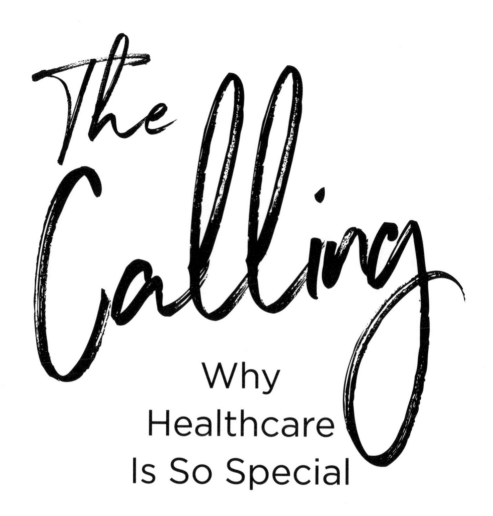

The Calling

Why Healthcare Is So Special

Quint Studer

Published by:
The Gratitude Group Publishing
220 West Garden St., Suite 501
Pensacola, FL 32502
www.thegratitudegroup.com

ISBN: 978-1-73707-890-6

Library of Congress Control Number: 2021938044

The stories in this book are true. However, some names and identifying details have been changed to protect the privacy of all concerned.

Printed in the United States of America

For every copy of *The Calling* purchased, The Gratitude Group Publishing will donate $1 to each of the following causes/organizations:

AUPHA Teaching Excellence in Health Administration Fund

AUPHA is a global network of colleges, universities, faculty, individuals, and organizations dedicated to the improvement of health and healthcare delivery through excellence in healthcare management and policy education. Its mission is to foster excellence and drive innovation in health management and policy education, and promote the value of university-based management education for leadership roles in the health sector. For more information, please visit www.aupha.org.

American College of Healthcare Executives (ACHE) Fund for Healthcare Leadership

The Fund for Healthcare Leadership provides scholarships to robust programs that inspire tomorrow's leaders. Scholarships are designed for those whose organizations may lack the resources to fully fund their tuition. Scholarships are provided for ACHE's executive programs that invite healthcare leaders to learn, share, and grow together. For more information, please visit www.ache.org.

The DAISY Foundation

The DAISY Foundation expresses gratitude to nurses with programs that recognize them for the extraordinary, skillful, compassionate care they provide patients and families. Our expression of gratitude will help nurses always remember the unforgettable impact their care has on patients and families, inspiring nurses to provide extraordinary care not only with their brains but also with their hearts. For more information, please visit www.daisyfoundation.org.

A Note to Readers

My books are written so that each chapter can be a standalone. The stories and information are self-contained. One does not necessarily need the rest of the book to understand a single chapter. I do this for I know how full each of your days are.

This way people can pull out specific chapters for development. It's easier to utilize the information if all content relevant to the topic is grouped in the same chapter.

As a result, cover-to-cover readers will see that certain tactics are repeated in more than one place—the same tactic with a tweak for a different outcome. People are reintroduced in the stories (titles and so forth) as a convenience to the reader. It saves time by not having to flip to another chapter.

Thank you for reading this book. I wish you all the best on your journey to fulfill your calling. I am grateful to each of you.

"A heart full of gratitude has little room for anything else."

—Quint Studer

Table of Contents

Introduction

Years ago, I wrote lyrics to a song. Acclaimed musician and songwriter Alex Call, along with the amazing singer Lisa Carrie, took these lyrics into a Nashville studio, made them much better, and put music to them. The lyrics we collaborated on went on to become the song "The Calling." Here's how it goes:

The Calling
(Quint Studer, Alex Call)

I'm not sure when it sparked, the fire deep inside
That made me want to make a difference
To touch others' lives
Was it when the nurse wiped away my tears, the time the doctor
    helped me overcome my fears
Like a seed it slowly grew
Until I knew

The calling
Was calling me
And I could hear it
The calling
Was calling me

THE CALLING

At first it was like a distant whisper
The message was unclear
But as time went by
It got so it was all that I could hear

The calling
Was calling me
And I could hear it
The calling
Was calling me

Woah, woah, woah
The calling
To the calling
Woah, woah, woah
The calling

I began to see little miracles, connections of the heart
I began to see how fires can grow from a single compassionate
    spark

The calling
Was calling me
And I could hear it
The calling
Was calling me
In my soul
The calling
Was calling me
I could hear it
The calling
Was calling me

Following my inner voice
I have no regrets at all
I just thank God I was listening when I got the call

I'm not sure when it sparked, the fire deep inside
That made me want to make a difference
To touch others' lives

Woah, woah, woah
The calling
I can hear it
Woah, woah, woah
The calling
In my soul
Woah, woah, woah
The calling
I can hear it calling me
Woah, woah, woah
The calling
I can hear the calling
Oh, can you hear it
In your spirit[1]

Now for the story of how this song came to be. I was speaking in Nashville, and like I always did, I made a comment about music. At the end of the day, I met Lisa Carrie, who had attended the workshop. In addition to working in healthcare, she is a very accomplished singer. She has an album produced by Andrew Gold, who was a member of Linda Ronstadt's band. She was a backup singer for artists like Eddy Arnold, Wayne Newton, Mickey Gilley and Gilley's Urban Cowboy Band, and Charlie Louvin on the Grand Ole Opry. As we talked music, I shared that I often thought of potential song lyrics. She encouraged me to send some her way. I did.

About three months later, I received a note from Lisa. Her partner at the time, Alex Call, had put music to these lyrics. If you aren't familiar with Alex Call, he was with the band Clover. He was a guitar player and lead singer. The harmonica player and backup singer was a fellow named Huey Lewis. The lead guitar player was John McFee, the lead guitar player for the Doobie Brothers. When Clover broke up, Alex continued to write music and play. He still does. Two of his best-known songs are "Little Too Late," which he wrote for Pat Benatar, and "867-5309/Jenny," written for Tommy Tutone. It was a rush to hear my lyrics performed by Alex.

Then, Alex wrote that my lyrics were not bad, and if I had others, to please send them his way. So I did. He, Lisa, and Michael Black and Gary Pigg, who are longtime Nashville musicians, recorded an entire CD. We called it *Passion & Purpose*.

One of the songs on the album is "Time to Live." While doing the recording, Lisa was diagnosed with breast cancer. After aggressive treatment, she is cancer-free. The lyrics to this song, which she wrote, address the impact of the diagnosis and the clarity of a time to live.

Another song was "The Calling" and you just read its lyrics above. It is about people answering the calling to make a difference. It is still a thrill to get a note that an organization played it at orientation or a school played it for graduation.

I've met thousands of people in healthcare. What all people in healthcare have in common is a great desire to be helpful and useful. People enter healthcare with a full emotional bank account. They are excited to enter such a great profession. The calling applies to everyone: providers, clinical staff, non-clinicians, and healthcare leaders and managers. Everyone works together with the goal of providing the best possible care to patients.

Many have spent years in school to prepare for their role. Those whose specific job did not require schooling in healthcare still are excited to be part of healthcare. These individuals may work in environmental services, finance, human resources, facilities, engineering, security, patient transporters, and medical assistants, to name a few. What all people also have in common is being excited to have a job in healthcare—the opportunity to do purposeful and worthwhile work and make a difference.

I ask people, "When you got your first job in healthcare, whom did you tell?" The answer is usually "my family" or "everyone." The challenge is to build on the excitement of that first job.

One goal of this book is to help readers who have a full emotional bank account to keep it, and to help those who don't have a full bank account to fill it back up. Hopefully, the book will provide some "deposits" for you. Another goal of this book is to provide tools and techniques that will be helpful (or make you feel good for already using these tools and techniques). The final goal is to help people identify and remove or decrease obstacles that block us from achieving our desired outcomes. These are barriers that have gotten in my way and at times still do.

This book is a labor of love. It's similar to the first book I ever wrote, *Hardwiring Excellence*, which came out in 2003. At first back then I didn't know if I could even write a book. It's hard. It is much easier for me to get up and speak than to write. I don't spell well, and grammar is not my strength. I wrote that book because of what a person said to me at a talk.

This person said to me, "There are many people who are not able to come hear you talk, but who could really benefit from the material."

It is my hope that the same is true for this book. I want it to be helpful and useful. *The Calling* will touch on things I've learned from my experiences as well as watching many others in healthcare. It will encompass many things I've learned since 2016, which I'll explain as we move along.

Healthcare people work too hard not to feel good about what they do. Healthcare workers have perfectionism in their DNA. There's always that internal battle between getting better and being perfect. There are times when being better, while not perfect, is important and needed, and times, of course, when perfection is a must. Due to the important work being done, healthcare workers tend to be very hard on themselves. We take home what did not work versus what did go well.

Healthcare is an emotional roller coaster. We go up and down because the work we do goes up and down. One minute we can be saving a life, and the next minute we can be telling someone that they're losing a loved one. One minute we can feel great about ourselves and management. The next minute we can feel like we're just not good at all. There's a time when you feel you've done a great job, and then there are those times when you feel you could do better.

When people ask me for advice, the starting point is always "Be kind to yourself." There are enough challenges in healthcare coming from other sources that can wear us down without our beating ourselves up. In healthcare, we're trained to notice what's wrong way more than what's right. And while that is valid and valuable in many cases, it is not always helpful when it comes to maintaining one's morale.

One of the hardest things to do in healthcare is to have a person accept a compliment. Just try it. Go compliment someone and you may find they actually push back a little bit. They'll say, "Well, I could do better." Or, "Well, I wish I would have done this sooner." Or, "I try." It's almost like they don't feel comfortable receiving a compliment.

In my 30s, I hit an emotional wall and started therapy. During a session, the therapist shared what she was observing. She told me when she gave me positive feedback, I rejected it by my words and body language. I turned away. When she gave me more constructive or less-than-positive feedback, I accepted it. Her conclusion was that one of the reasons I felt so depressed was I filter out the positive and let in only the negative. Many of us in healthcare do that. I hope this book helps you let in the positive. You work too hard not to feel great about what you do.

This book is about keeping the emotional bank account full and filling it back up. When you read it, I want you to laugh a little bit. You may shed a tear here and there.

My message to those reading this book is this: You're going to hopefully read things you are doing already and learnings that can be helpful and useful to you. A great trait of those who work in healthcare is the drive to be the best one can be. We want to look at how we can be better at what we do because the impact is so vital.

Healthcare is loaded with people who have answered the calling. They didn't get into healthcare for money. They didn't get into healthcare for a balanced life. They didn't get into healthcare for easy work hours. They were called into healthcare by their strong desire to be helpful and useful. And that's what I hope this book is for you.

I dedicate this book to you who answer the calling every day and make the impossible possible. I have such admiration for you. I am grateful for the difference you make.

CHAPTER 1

The Calling Is in Our DNA

I entered healthcare later in life, which is unusual. I was in my early thirties. When I say "the calling," I mean that people who choose to work in healthcare answered a calling. It happens for some sooner than others; however, there always exists a pull inside each person to be part of something that makes a positive difference.

I ask people, "When did you first start thinking about healthcare?"

When I ask nurses when they first thought about nursing as a career, they usually say it happened very early. People say they were a nurse on Halloween when they were a child. They loved to play hospital. They had one of those medical bags from years ago with all the equipment needed to pretend they were a doctor or a nurse.

When asked the same thing, physicians usually say they had the calling early on and certainly by college. I ask them why they chose to be a doctor. I say, "Did you go to a website and start looking at compensation?" And they laugh and say no, that wasn't it at all. They just felt a real desire to make a difference. Often they didn't know exactly what type of doctor they were going to be, but they *did* know they wanted to be a doctor. And then in medical school they would do a rotation and something would click. They'd realize "this is what I want to do."

I met the first female urologist in a large, well-known healthcare system and asked her why she chose urology. It seems the field chose her as much as she chose it. She said she wanted to be an internal medicine specialist as it would let her get to know her patients on a longer-term basis. She also really loved surgery. And as she was going through rotations, the urology rotation clicked. She saw that this was the best of both worlds.

It's not only clinicians who have the market cornered on this sense of calling. Everyone in healthcare has this calling. For example, there is a CPA who performed an audit of a healthcare system. He was attracted to how he felt when he was there and ended up working in their finance department.

Think of people who work in information technology, food services, human resources, environmental services, facilities engineering, security, and so forth in a healthcare setting. In many of these roles, a person could work anywhere. They could have better hours and a better balance of life and not deal with the emotions that are part of healthcare. Yet they chose healthcare. These individuals answered the same calling as clinicians. In fact, if you're a clinician, you're probably going to work in healthcare, but if you're not, you certainly made a deliberate choice in choosing this field.

Over the years, I've heard story after story about such individuals making a huge impact on people's lives. For example, I was working with a healthcare organization, and Jeff Atwood was one of the key leaders. We still communicate. Jeff has written some wonderful books on children and leadership. He and his wife knew there were going to be some challenges in their oldest daughter's development due to special needs (which I also call special gifts). They were very nervous. She had been critically ill early in her life, and of course they were searching for the best answers possible. They went to a very well-respected medical center with a large children's hospital.

They parked and walked into this large, imposing building. On the way in, they walked past a parking lot attendant. This family was from a smaller community and was accustomed to smaller hospitals. Because of that and the emotional nature of the whole situation, both Jeff and his wife were rather overwhelmed by everything that was going on. They were questioning everything, including whether they were in the right place for their daughter. As Jeff was walking to get the car after the appointment, the parking lot attendant they had encountered earlier stopped him and said, "I just want you to know that while you've been in there, I've been praying for you."

As they got in their car, they took that interaction as a sign they were in the right place. And as you know, reducing anxiety and replacing it with the feeling they're in the right place is huge to a patient and their family.

Just think if that parking lot attendant had worked in a parking garage that wasn't attached to a hospital. If you came out of a mall and the attendant said, "While you've been shopping, I've been praying for you," it may not have quite the same impact as it did at this medical center! But that parking lot attendant who could work anywhere chose to work in a hospital. You will likely agree that they are helpful and useful.

Here is another story that resonates with me. The story happened when I was speaking in Peoria.

Before speaking to groups of employees, I would ask managers to share a note or story about an employee they knew was coming to one of these sessions. I would tell managers, "I can't promise I'll mention all of the stories but will try my best to do so." A manager of a nursing and labor-delivery unit wrote a note about a person in food services. The employee didn't report to her, yet she wanted to make sure I knew how valuable this person was. One of the food service worker's jobs was passing out trays. Her note told of a very young mother without any support who had come to the hospital and delivered a stillborn child.

My first grandchild was a stillborn birth, and my son and daughter-in-law were given time to be with their daughter, Ella, to say goodbye. As they do, the hospital gave this mom time to be with her baby to say goodbye, at least physically. The mother was alone and had no support system. Knowing this organization, I guarantee you that doctors, pastoral care, nurses, and social workers all offered to be with this young mother, but she said no. She said she didn't need them to be with her.

Around that time, the trays were starting to be passed out. The lady passing out the trays calmly knocked on the door and walked in and immediately realized what she had come upon. And she said to the young mother, "I'm so sorry. I know you want to be alone." The mother looked at the food service person passing out the trays and said, "No, I don't." So the food service worker sat down on the bed with the young mom. The mother asked her big questions like, "Why did this happen? How can I tell people?" And the tray passer answered all of her questions. You see, she saw a chance to be helpful and useful, and she took it.

You might wonder why the young mom didn't take the offering of help from the other people in the hospital. My guess is she just felt more comfortable with the food service worker. And in the note the nurse manager wrote she said, "When she came to work today, she thought she was going to be passing out trays, which is an important job. But today she did more than that. She passed out love."

Again…somebody in food service could probably work anywhere. I am just in awe of everyone who chooses to work in the healthcare environment. That's the calling. That's what this book is about: how we can continue to ignite our own flame, rekindle our own passion for this work, and help others to do the same. As employee motivation and engagement expert Dr. Bob Nelson says, "You get the best effort from others not by lighting a fire beneath them, but by building a fire within."

Each of us has a fire inside of us. Sometimes our fire almost gets put out. Notice the word "almost." I believe that fire can be rekindled, and that it will burn for as long as we live. And our fire will help others ignite their internal fire.

Certainly, there are cold winds blowing constantly in healthcare, whether it's a pandemic, the challenge of different payer mixes, dealing with mergers and consolidations, facing new competition that pops up, or staff shortages. There's probably never been a time in healthcare where we can say it was just smooth sailing. Now it might seem like that looking in the rearview mirror, but while we were in it, it was always choppy water. And some waves are much choppier than others.

But if we look at stories like these, we can clearly see that the one thing that's been constant is that each and every day, people keep coming out to do the best they can to make the organization they work with the best it can be. They have to. It's in their DNA.

CHAPTER 2

My Own Healthcare Calling

We all have our own story about how we came to be in healthcare. Please allow me to share my story. I think it will help explain where I'm coming from.

I started out as a teacher for children with special needs. I went to Lyons Township High School. It's a large high school in La Grange, Illinois. While there, I played soccer. If you have read my books or heard me speak, you may have heard about Coach King, who had a big impact on my life.

Back in 1969, as a senior I had two study halls. If you had two study halls, you could get released from one, but you had to have a good reason to get out of it. So Coach King let me come into his classroom and be what you might call a teacher assistant. I helped with his students who had special needs. My job was to walk his male students to the library after the bell rang, sit with them until right before the bell rang again, and then walk them back to the classroom.

This took place at a time when education was making the first attempts at mainstreaming. In other words, people with special needs were not placed in separate schools, but "mainstreamed" as much as possible into the regular school and classrooms. Back then (and, sadly, probably even today), these were kids who would sometimes get teased and called names. The hope was that by walking with them and sitting with them, I would help prevent that from happening. I enjoyed doing this; in fact, it was the highlight of my day.

I went to college at the University of Wisconsin-Whitewater. There weren't a lot of college degrees in my family, but my parents were determined that I go to college. So off I went to college, with no idea of what to study.

At the end of my sophomore year, my academic advisor informed me that it was time to pick a major in order to graduate on time. So we talked about majors, and I thought about people who had an impact on my life. I realized it was teachers, particularly Coach King, who had made that kind of impact. And so I told him I wanted to be a teacher. It would be neat to be in a high school. I like that environment. I like the pep rallies. I love sports.

Then he said, "What type of teacher?" And I got very concerned. I have grammar issues and spelling issues, and what can you teach if you can't spell and write very well? Then it just hit me that I really liked what Coach King did back at Lyons Township. So I explained about Coach King, and the counselor said, "Oh, you want to be a teacher for children with special needs."

With that, I became a teacher for these wonderful kids. It was a job I really loved. I felt useful and helpful, and enjoyed that time in my life very, very much. I didn't know at the time how much of my training I would still use today. There are so many parallels. In this arena, a parent feels their child may not be developing as expected so they seek an assessment. Based on the results, a plan is developed to maximize the child's potential. The person who interacts with each child understands their role and responsibility to help the child, and so they adjust treatment as needed. This approach also works in life and work: diagnose, plan, treat, and adjust.

This is where fate stepped in. If you look back over your own life, you will see there's a person who made a huge difference. Maybe it was a parent, or a community member, or a leader, or a coworker—someone impacted your life in a way that reshaped your future. If that hadn't happened, you might have turned a different direction—not a wrong one, just a different one. For me, it was Coach King. It was his influence that made me a teacher, and for that I'm so grateful.

While things were going well, one of my personal challenges was mental health issues. I struggle with depression, and for years thought I could solve my depression with a drink. In December of 1982, I woke up one morning and it hit me that drinking wasn't helping. In fact, it was hurting. People call it hitting rock bottom. It's also called a moment of clarity. While I had not lost a job, I had lost my family and certainly my self-respect. I entered the world of addiction recovery.

I've been in recovery ever since that December day in 1982.

As part of recovery, I would go to a local treatment hospital for twelve-step meetings. During this time, the hospital was bought by Lutheran General Health System via an entity called Parkside Medical Services Corporation. I read that Parkside was looking for someone to work in community relations. I gave the listed number a call. Their corporate office was in Park Ridge, Illinois.

This is where fate pops in once again. Orville McElfresh, their vice president of marketing, answered the phone. And the reason he answered is because the assistant happened to be gone. Normally I wouldn't have gotten Orville McElfresh. But on this day I did. I told him a little bit about myself: that I worked in education, had helped set up a student assistance program for the school district where I was living for children raised in alcoholic families, and so on. And he said, "Why don't you send me a résumé?"

Not being unhappy in my current job, I hung up thinking I would not pursue the job. I rationalized that I was fine. I also had a fear of failure and was afraid I wasn't going to get the job.

A little while later, Orville McElfresh called and he said, "We've got somebody coming up to Wisconsin, and if you're available, I'd love for him to meet with you." We met and I became a community relations coordinator for Parkside Lodge of Wisconsin, which was a 35-bed drug and alcohol hospital (19 beds for adults and 16 beds for adolescents).

That's the story of how I got into healthcare. And I loved it. While I always felt helpful and useful as a teacher for children with special needs, as a recovering alcoholic, I was particularly drawn to that feeling of being involved and seeing patients and families be put back together. Of course, there was also the downside that comes with any type of healthcare that provides care to people who don't achieve the desired outcome. But the work was so rewarding.

Part of the job was calling on businesses, usually human resources professionals. At the time, drug and alcohol addiction were getting significant attention, so I could usually get in the door and share with them the services we offered.

It is common practice when an employee leaves treatment to have a "back-to-work" session between the counselor, the patient, their supervisor, and someone from human resources. They discuss how this employee is going to come back into the workplace, what to look for, what would happen if the person doesn't follow through with the treatment and recovery. Going to these sessions led to my meeting many human resources professionals.

One of the places I went was Mercy Hospital, in Janesville, Wisconsin. The human resources director was Bea Hedding. One day she said, "We're adding a new position here called the director of marketing. You do a good job in community relations, and we are wondering if you would like to consider being our director of marketing."

Now, I was in that state of not knowing what I don't know. So I said, "I'd love that!" The thought was, *Wow, if we do great stuff for people with drug and alcohol problems, wouldn't it be neat to work in a hospital that treats people with all sorts of other issues?* This was a big employer and it was exciting. My dad was pretty pumped about my being a director at a large organization.

I soon realized I had no idea what I was doing. Like most organizations back then, they didn't have a robust training and development program. So I just started going out and reading and studying on my own. The biggest impact on me was Tom Peters and Robert H. Waterman's book *In Search of Excellence.*

This led to my working there for a little over six years, eventually being senior vice president of business development. And again, that serendipity happened. Tom Giella who was with a search firm called. He mentioned there was a job in Chicago he wanted to talk to me about. I was relatively happy with where I was. He said, "Well, I'm going to be up in Janesville because I have relatives there. Why don't we get together for a cup of coffee?" So we did and he said he'd really like me to go meet Mark Clement, who was the new president/CEO at Holy Cross Hospital in Chicago.

The job seemed like a lateral move to me. But Tom encouraged me to make the trip, so I went down and talked to Mark, and it turned out to be a great gift. We talked about my strengths and where more development was needed. And then he offered me a job at Holy Cross as the senior vice president. In essence, I was the chief operating officer. It changed my life. I learned so much from Mark, as he is a role model leader.

It turned out to be a wonderful job for a surprising reason: Our hospital didn't have a lot of money, so we had to be creative. And that's where I was introduced to patient experience. In fact, I was put in charge of it. My Holy Cross experience is detailed in *Hardwiring Excellence*. The three years there were like a residency in leadership development, employee engagement, physician engagement, and patient experience. It was a time for trying things. Mark taught us to be okay with progress versus perfection.

If you've read my other books, you may know the story of how it went. We went from single-digit patient satisfaction to top-tier results. We ended up getting attention, and people started visiting us. And one of those visitors was from Baptist Hospital in Pensacola, Florida. They invited me to come down and tell the story. Then in March of 1996, Baptist offered me the administrative/president job at the large hospital, which also included a 50-bed facility called Gulf Breeze Hospital. So I came down to Pensacola with a goal to keep developing the tools, techniques, and processes, with a focus on consistency, reliability, and sustainability.

An observation over the years has been that everyone in a healthcare entity can be really great at moments, but is there consistency? If so, how do you sustain it? It seems we put so much effort into making improvements; however, holding and growing the gains can be difficult. Due to the external environment, if we stay the same, we go backwards. Healthcare can feel like walking up an escalator that is going down. It requires constant improvement.

Like any situation, it was three steps forward and two steps back. Building on past experience and adding systems to hardwire the tools, techniques, and processes, Baptist Hospital achieved very high performance. During this time, the Health Care Advisory Board completed a study on patient satisfaction. Holy Cross and Baptist were prominently mentioned. This led to many healthcare colleagues visiting Baptist and asking me to present to their organizations, which in turn led to the start of Studer Group® in 2000.

Studer Group started out with my wife (Rishy), myself, and Sheila Martin, who had been my secretary at Baptist Hospital. And we had a $15,000 engagement. After working so hard to become a president of a hospital, now I was leaving that job for the unknown. I was leaving a great organization, people I loved, a great salary, benefits, and a pension program. Plus, there was still that internal fear of failure.

When I walked out of Baptist, I was a nervous wreck. I almost didn't do it. But Norm Adams, who was a spiritual advisor of mine, met with me. He talked to me about how sometimes our heart gets aroused, and when that happens, we should follow it. Making a change might not provide the security of where we are at the time, but we lose opportunities if we don't go where our hearts are aroused. It's really about following your passion.

So we started Studer Group. We met wonderful people. Studer Group's mission was to make healthcare better for patients to receive care, employees to work, and physicians to practice medicine. Our vision was to help people and organizations achieve their maximum potential.

It was quite a ride. At first, so many saw what we did as "soft" or people skills. To me, they are the essential skills. We were constantly learning alongside those organizations we were working with. While the work was about getting better, it's important to link back to what is right in healthcare. Every day we saw people doing incredible work, work that had purpose, was worthwhile, and made a difference. The work eventually led to Studer Group's earning the Malcolm Baldrige National Quality Award in 2010.

We also had many employees looking for opportunities for growth, and we were not the biggest company. There are many bigger companies, and employees were going to be limited with us. And so Studer Group was eventually sold to Huron Consulting Group in 2015.

In any strategic sale, there will be changes and challenges, but you go in with your eyes wide open. I stayed with Huron for a year after it acquired Studer Group until I felt the time was right for me to resign. I knew that I had a five-year non-healthcare non-compete; however, at the time, it did not seem like a big deal. It was not long after leaving that I realized how much I underestimated the impact leaving healthcare would have on me psychologically.

You may have heard the story that when surgeons retire, they don't have a long life after that. It's just so hard, because so much of your life is put into making a difference, and while you can make a difference in other ways, all of a sudden you have this void. That's what happened. For the first two years after leaving Huron, I struggled mightily. I had stomachaches and headaches and went to doctors and mental health therapists to be treated for issues like fear and depression. It was very, very difficult.

Fortunately, throughout that time, I had gotten very involved in the local community and started doing many, many activities to revitalize Pensacola. I had started a not-for-profit called the Better Pensacola Forum, which later became Studer Community Institute (SCI). This led to some wonderful things. SCI has three main focuses: 1) early brain development, which leads to kindergarten readiness and good school performance, which in turn helps create a strong talent base, 2) workforce training and development because most jobs are local and economic development is a cornerstone of vibrancy, and 3) civic engagement, because civic IQ determines whether a citizen will buy into initiatives and drive them forward. You can learn more by visiting www.studeri.org.

What saved me the most was serving on boards and some lifelines people gave me. I was fortunate to be asked to serve on the board of

Ascension Sacred Heart Health System by Susan Davis, who at the time was its president and CEO. It was an honor to be a part of the building of the new children's hospital at Sacred Heart. It was an incredibly fulfilling experience at a time when I needed to feel useful and helpful again.

Another lifeline came from Mark Clement of TriHealth, Cincinnati, Ohio. He asked me to serve on the TriHealth Board of Trustees and the Bethesda Inc. Board of Trustees. Mark must have known I needed this. As he has been since 1993, Mark was there when I needed him. TriHealth and Bethesda are world-class organizations. Hazelden Betty Ford Foundation provided the next lifeline. I was asked to serve on their board. I have always been in awe of Hazelden Betty Ford. While I always thought they were special, being a board member confirmed it.

The next two lifelines were AUPHA (the Association of University Programs in Health Administration) and CAHME (the Commission on Accreditation of Healthcare Management Education).

I served on the board of AUPHA for many years. In fact, a door prize for their national conference was that I would go to affiliated colleges and speak to their classes. That really was wonderful. I met so many great people. I've stayed in touch with AUPHA and love the work they do. Dan Gentry, their CEO and president, and I are close. Through his help, every couple of weeks I'm a guest lecturer at some university in the area of healthcare administration. I truly enjoy that.

My friend Anthony Stanowski, president and CEO of CAHME, put me on their board. CAHME is the accrediting body for healthcare management graduate programs in the U.S. and Canada. It has been really marvelous to be on that board because it's kept me engaged in healthcare.

So I've been very fortunate to be affiliated with these fine organizations.

Finally, I am grateful to present each year to healthcare students at many colleges and universities.

During my time away from healthcare, I wrote two books. One was *Building a Vibrant Community*, which was published in 2018. By "vibrant community," I mean one that has a thriving economy and all the features that make young people want to stay home or come back to after college. As Jim Clifton says in *The Coming Jobs War*, it's all about talent. Capital follows talent, but talent follows place. So vibrant communities are great places for people to work and live.

Then in 2020, came *The Busy Leader's Handbook*. It features 41 best practices learned during my career, particularly those I've learned since 2016 while dealing with so many small businesses as part of my not-for-profit institute. Also, I have such a heart for middle managers. Like many people, I didn't go the MHA or MBA route. Ninety percent of what I learned was from on-the-job training. *The Busy Leader's Handbook* is really a reference guide for middle managers. And best of all, I've been able to use it in my work inside communities as they build up their local businesses.

So these have been some exciting times. I'm even more excited about the book you're reading now than I have been about a book in the past 16 or 17 years. I now know what it's like to be able to live your calling. And I also know what it's like to not be able to live your calling, so it's even more heartfelt to write a book dedicated to those working in healthcare.

These last five years have been a gift. They taught me an awful lot about myself. Now I've reached that point of being very excited to have the opportunity to potentially be useful once again in healthcare.

In the recovery community, I talk all the time about how we're the lucky ones. Somebody with an addiction normally ends up in one of three places: in recovery, in jail, or dead. Sadly, so many of them end up in the latter two situations. The lucky ones are those of us who got that moment of clarity. We got to hold up the mirror and turn our lives around, which made us better human beings and better members of the human race as long as we help others.

We in healthcare are lucky too. We can do what we love full-time. It's typical for people in healthcare to do volunteer work in something that also is a helpful, useful thing. Maybe it's at their school, their community, or their church. One of my favorite topics is what people do when they retire. Many times they try to do what they did while working, but they do it for free. They volunteer at a free clinic, for example.

One time I asked Bubba Watson, who is a professional golfer and my business partner in many things here in Pensacola, what he was going to do when he retired. The first thing he said is golf. Why? Because he loves golf! This makes a lot of sense.

When speaking to students, the most asked question is, "What's your biggest career advice?" I tell them: "Pick something you love, something you're passionate about, because every job will have times that are tough. Every job is going to have a moment or two when we want to quit. If we love what we're doing, we're going to get through those tough, tough times. If we don't love it, we're not."

We're fortunate for the most part in healthcare that we can do what we're passionate about. We can get paid at a rate that allows us to do it full-time. So I've often said we're the lucky ones, and truly believe that. I hope as you contemplate your career—where you are now and where you're going—that you also realize you're one of the lucky ones.

We get to do something we feel passionate about every day, and we get to make a living doing it. Life doesn't get much better than that.

CHAPTER 3

Leadership Is an Inside Job

"When the student is ready, the teacher will appear."
—Attributed to The Buddha, Lao Tzu, and the Theosophists

Leadership is an inside job. However, that inside job may be sparked or helped along by many, many outside voices.

Over the years, many great books have been written.

For example, I loved Sheldon Bowles and Ken Blanchard's book *Gung Ho!* and Spencer Johnson, MD's *Who Moved My Cheese?* It seemed for a while in healthcare everybody was reading *Who Moved My Cheese?* These are still excellent books.

There are also those books and authors who have been around for decades. Here, I think of authors like Peter Drucker and W. Edwards Deming. Other examples are Tom Peters and Robert H. Waterman's book *In Search of Excellence.* Another one is Sun Tzu's *The Art of War.* For years, that was a go-to book for most anyone in leadership in any arena.

As an entrepreneur-in-residence at the University of West Florida, I have everybody read *The E-Myth Revisited* by Michael E. Gerber. It's a great book if you're an entrepreneur or starting a company. Certainly, Jim Collins' *Good to Great* has been one of those books that have had lasting power. I loved *Built to Last* by Collins even more than *Good to Great*, but that's my own taste.

There are books today that stay on the bestseller list year after year, like *StrengthsFinder 2.0* by Tom Rath. *StrengthsFinder* was originally introduced by Gallup in the 2001 book *Now, Discover Your Strengths*. I have huge respect for Gallup and its CEO and chairman, Jim Clifton. I often think about the number of people Gallup and its books have helped over the years. I can only hope my writings have a fraction of this kind of lasting power.

There are many, many tools and resources one can utilize to be the best they can be, and books are some of my favorite. Often it is the second or third time I read a book that it sinks in. You have to be ready to hear and receive it. I've said many times, "When the student is ready, the teacher will appear." If you will look at the top of this chapter, you'll see that this is a famous quote that has been attributed to many different individuals.

I used to say when I heard or read something, "I have never heard that before." It turns out that more often than not, I *have* heard it or read it—I just was not ready to learn it. It calls to mind another quote, this one by Samuel Johnson: "People need to be reminded more often than they need to be instructed."

This became clear when a person mentioned something in a presentation and I went up to him and said, "Wow. I loved that. Where did you learn that?" He said, "It's in this book." I said, "This is unbelievable. I have that book. Where is it in that book?" He told me it was on page 83, and I said, "You're kidding. I've never read that."

Then I pulled the book out. I had read it, yellow-marked it, underlined it, and pink-marked it. In fact, I had read it three times and still had not remembered it. Somehow, though, based on where I was in my life and also at that moment, it suddenly made a heck of a lot of sense. So, when the student is ready, the teacher appears.

It means as a teacher and a leader, I needed to deflate my ego. It also means that I may not be the teacher, even for people who report to me. It's really hard when somebody says they've never heard something before and I know I've already told them. The lesson was to not take it personally. One cannot control where other people are in their journey of learning.

When I was administrator at Baptist Hospital in Pensacola, Florida, an author came to speak to the leadership team. He talked about how to increase employee engagement.

When he finished speaking, he received a well-earned standing ovation. I was excited they liked him so much, but was also probably a little jealous. Envy gets in the way at times; however, I am so much better now—time does that. I approached one of our leaders, a manager, and asked her how she liked it. She said, "I didn't like it; I loved it!"

I asked, "What did you love?" She said, "Well, this part. I've never heard this before." It was a tip the speaker had given on how to show them you care. I thought to myself, *Well, you have heard it before—I've said it before. In fact, I've said it at department meetings before.*

Now, being a rather immature person at the time (and probably still today), I wanted to demonstrate to her that I had said it first. So, I thought, *How can I do this? Should I bring somebody over and say, "Do you remember when I said this?"* Then it hit me. *You know what? It doesn't matter. What's important is it sunk in now!* When the student is ready, the teacher appears. (This was also a good reminder that great leaders care more about results being achieved than about who gets credit for those results.)

Earlier we covered how little we read and hear is new. Most of it has been said before, by someone else, somewhere. And that's okay. It's okay to say it again, your way, and put your own twist on it. Maybe your way will resonate with someone.

In fact, in many cases, it's really not the innovator who scales something. It's the imitator. I wrote an article on why we need to be grateful for the imitators. They're not copycats. We should always give credit if other people's intellectual capital is involved, of course, but often we can take an idea someone had, or a product they invented, and figure out how to increase its use and impact. Many times, this happens across industries: One industry makes a discovery, but it's another industry that figures out how to scale it or use it in a different way.

It feels good when someone take a tool or technique I introduced and makes it better. In addition, to see how others are using technology to make accessing resources to help people working in healthcare is thrilling. The goal was and still is to help patients receive better care, provide employees a better place to work, and provide physicians a better place to practice medicine.

There are an abundance of tools, techniques, and practices that we in healthcare can implement at different times, as we are always striving to get better. We will look at some of these as we go through this book. First, though, let's start off with those things that at times get in the way of achieving our desired results. When the student is ready, the teacher will appear.

In December of 1982, with that moment of clarity that a drink won't help, I became teachable. All of a sudden, things I'd been hearing finally clicked. I could go to therapy and really maximize what I had heard or read. I learned to stop blaming the therapist or other people and circumstances in my life.

In *The Busy Leader's Handbook*, the first chapter is the key to everything that follows. It's titled "Strive to Be Self-Aware and Coachable." If a person doesn't have self-awareness, it's over. They're not going to know what they're good at, but mostly, they're not going to know what they can improve upon. There's a variety of techniques in that book on how to improve self-awareness. Once aware, we are more coachable. This means being willing to listen and implement the lessons.

Harry Gruner is founder and managing general partner of JMI Equity. I have great respect for Harry. We had breakfast one morning and I asked him, "Harry, when you look at investing in a company, how do you make the decision?"

I thought he'd say things like, "Well, can you raise prices? What's the runway?" (Meaning, what is the growth opportunity?) He told me how many companies they'd looked at to possibly invest in, which was in the hundreds; how many they'd then dug deep into, which was way, way fewer; and how many they would invest in, which was maybe two or three a year. I asked him how he made those decisions, and he said, "There are two main drivers: self-awareness and coachability of the founder."

He explained that his firm isn't investing in a company to keep it the same. They're investing in the company to grow it. If a founder is stuck on saying, "Here's how this company has to run," they might not be coachable enough to adjust to some of the recommendations that they will receive.

So, in the spirit of self-awareness and coachability, we'll spend the next several chapters walking through a presentation that I have given in the last couple of years.

The theme of that presentation, and the next section of this book, is that leadership starts as an inside job. Sometimes progress is made not by reading that next book, or talking to that next consultant, or hearing that next lecture, or trying that newest tool. These things can help. However, real growth happens when we get rid of stuff that blocks us from maximizing the tools we already have, the leader we're already working with, the book we've already read, the consultant we've already heard.

When we get the inside right, the outside follows.

SECTION 2

The Barriers

This book is based on the belief that healthcare people are passionate about being helpful and useful. We all start our career with a full emotional bank account, and to truly answer the calling that led us to choose healthcare, we need to be sure we keep it full. As we travel through this book, we'll learn some ways to do that.

First, though, we need to address what it is that holds us back and blocks us from achieving our desired outcome.

One barrier we face is the scope and pace of change. There is so much to learn in healthcare: new procedures, systems, tools, and methods. These can overwhelm us and cause our human system to shut down. We cannot remove this barrier. Healthcare will always be defined by change. All we can do is learn to manage that change, and strive to keep getting better so we can meet the challenges it brings.

To do this, we need to focus on the barriers we *can* control. Some of these barriers are personal. They are psychological and emotional. Before we can get the outside things right and impact the growth of those around us, we need to get our insides right. Leadership is, first and foremost, an inside job.

The barriers that hold us back vary from person to person. Many of these personal barriers we may not be aware of at all. In fact, we may be more likely to recognize them in others before noticing them in ourselves! This is completely normal. Please do not feel bad about your barriers. They are basic human defense mechanisms. We all have them.

The other type of barrier is organizational. These are things we do (or don't do) that keep people from being the best they can be. We have touched on a few of these in this section of the book. People enter healthcare because they want to be helpful and useful. And if we can create a culture where they can be helpful and useful, that's really where the magic happens.

Getting intentional about recognizing and removing the barriers that get in our way and in the way of others is a game changer. It's what allows us to be as helpful and useful as we want to be—and as our coworkers and patients need us to be. Only then can we fully live up to our calling.

CHAPTER 4

Denial, Rationalization, and Blame

We will start this section with the most common barriers I see. I used to talk about these three barriers—denial, rationalization, and blame—independently. Now I combine them. That's because I have found that they are really intertwined.

Let's begin with denial. You've probably heard that denial is not a river in Africa. It's true. Denial is the river in our brain that keeps us from accepting the data and/or seeing things clearly. Too often, denial clicks in and blocks us from accepting our situation. For example, we may feel employee turnover is due only to compensation and benefits. However, there may be other reasons.

The challenge with denial is we don't know we're in it. Being a recovering alcoholic, I know denial well. And many times, the higher up one goes in leadership, the easier it is to be in denial. That's because fewer people are willing to challenge a supervisor. It's just a natural thing. Over the years, many, many leaders have said that one of the issues they all face is that people don't want to challenge them. I know that about me. While I don't want to shut off feedback, at times I do.

While we often don't want to hear it, it is the single best tool for breaking out of denial.

I have come up with my own techniques to assure I receive feedback. I ask people who work with me, "Help me now, am I going off the grid? What am I not thinking about?" If I don't ask, sometimes people will just hold back. Dr. Kevin Post, CMO of Avera Medical Group, says he has found it helpful to gather feedback by asking, "What is one thing I do or don't do that holds me back?" (That is why people in non-official supervisory roles can benefit from reading this book. Your manager needs your help. They need your feedback.)

A CEO told me she was frustrated that people didn't challenge her. I said, "You have a pretty strong personality. I could see where people could be a little intimidated by you." And she said, "Well, I'm not intimidating." I said, "I don't think people see themselves as intimidating, but sometimes it's the role."

Good leaders want feedback. The key is to create ways to make sure it happens. In fact, many times I will share with people to take a position they know doesn't make a lot of sense and see how long it takes for someone to question it. This lets you know if you have a culture that's mutually collaborative, trusting, and transparent, one where people are willing to give you the feedback you need to hear to get better and better. It's a journey.

One of the keys to overcoming denial is to surround ourselves with people who will provide us feedback, even when it's hard to hear. Beth Keane is a great example of a person who really got that concept. Beth passed away in 2013 from breast cancer. In 2013, I wrote the book *A Culture of High Performance*, which is dedicated to her. About three weeks before Beth passed away, I visited her at her house, and she was writing letters to grandchildren she would never meet, grandchildren who did not yet exist but whom she felt confident would be here someday. She wanted them to know who she was, her hopes, and love for them. That was the kind of person she was.

Beth was known for helping people have uncomfortable conversations, most notably the "Spinach in Your Teeth" message. Beth explained that when we love someone, we'll tell them they have spinach in their teeth. Her point was that giving someone an uncomfortable message is an act of caring.

It just seems to make a lot of sense. If I have shaving cream on my face, my wife will immediately tell me. I've walked out of hotels with shaving cream on my face. And I can't believe how many people I've talked to before someone finally says, "Hey, you've got shaving cream on your face," or, "Your button is unbuttoned," or, "Don't you realize your hair is sticking straight up?" (I've had people come up to me at speaking engagements when I'm on a break and actually start combing my hair!)

If you put "Beth Keane Spinach in Your Teeth" in the search bar, you will find her famous talk. It's a terrific teaching tool.

A big part of getting through denial is surrounding ourselves with people who will shoot straight with us. There are key things you might say, such as, "Please, I need your feedback. What have I said that doesn't ring well?"…or, "If you were an employee, how would you respond to this?"…or, "What can I do to make this better?"

Dick Fulford was one such person for me. Mr. Fulford and I worked together when I was administrator of Baptist Hospital in Pensacola. He officially reported to me. One day when I was holding a meeting with the senior team, it must have been obvious that I was filled with anxiety about the tough month we were having. I fell into the trap of complaining and blaming. Mr. Fulford called me out into the hallway and essentially told me to stop being so negative and defeatist. He said the others in the meeting were looking to me for confidence and support, not self-doubt. This must have been an uncomfortable message to share, but he cared enough to share it anyway. I adjusted, went back in and put his recommendation into practice. I apologized to the group and we discussed next steps.

Right now we are focused on denial, and shortly we're going to talk in more detail about rationalization and blame. But I'm going to also touch on those two barriers here because they can blend together. They're sort of like a gumbo. They swirl around in the same pot, some stronger than others at certain times.

Here's an example. I'm on social media, LinkedIn, and it's been gratifying to see people connect with me. I am grateful to hear stories about how they've used one of my books or heard me speak, etc. Recently, one hospital leader said, "Is there any way you could do a Zoom call with our leadership team? We're really depressed. The pandemic is wearing us down, and it'd be a great surprise if you could show up."

I said, "Of course," and added, "What else would you like?" And they said, "We really are frustrated because our HCAHPS results have really dropped." (HCAHPS, which stands for Hospital Consumer Assessment of Healthcare Providers and Systems, is a national standardized survey used to measure a patient's perception of care. It connects to reimbursement and makes it easier for patients to compare hospitals in areas they care about. HCAHPS questions cover areas like nurse communication, doctor communication, cleanliness, and so forth.)

This hospital is part of a huge system, and it was always one of the top hospitals in the system. But since COVID-19 began, it had dropped way, way back from being in the top 10 to the bottom 10. And of course they immediately jumped on the fact that it was COVID-19. This is where blame and rationalization come in.

The Zoom call went very well. It was very positive. But of course I had to do the spinach-in-your-teeth part by saying, "Well, everybody has COVID-19; you're not the only hospital. So the fact is you're in a system where you're compared to like hospitals in the system, the same corporate headquarters, the same everything else. So the key is to learn what others are doing that is working."

See? They were so focused on thinking nothing could be done due to the impact of COVID-19 they fell into the trap of denial, that "there's-nothing-we-can-do" feeling. That's the gumbo. That's how it all swirls together.

One final tip: A good way to help people move through denial (that nothing-can-be-done feeling) is to find success in the same organization. A group of people in a large medical center had overall results in HCAHPS that were low. They explained it was their lack of resources due to the poor payer mix. As the results were looked at more deeply, though, there were some areas with much better results than the others. They had the same payer mix and the same resources, yet better outcomes.

This technique starts to eliminate the "it-can't-be-done-here" mentality. Never underestimate what one area can do to show other areas ways to be better.

Rationalization Blocks the Best Solutions.

When we rationalize, we try to justify our actions (or lack of actions) by giving seemingly logical explanations for things that are actually based on other causes.

I am a master rationalizer. I tell people, "If you need to rationalize something, call me—I can help." It's a subconscious emotion. We do it because we believe it on some level. It makes sense. We are not able to recognize we are rationalizing. Like the other barriers, rationalizing keeps us from taking the best action we can take to turn the dial in whatever metric we're trying to achieve.

To combat rationalization, we need to relate versus compare. You know healthcare, we love to compare, which makes sense most of the time. We have productivity, FTE counts, cost per adjusted occupied bed, how long it takes somebody to get an appointment, and turnaround time—hundreds of measures. These are all vital. I'm a measurement person. But it's more effective if we look at these measurements and say, "Oh wow, they're better than us. Let's find out how they are doing it," versus coming up with why you are different from them and can't do better. When we do the latter, we end up in what I call "terminal uniqueness."

Patient experience is a good example. For a while, people would say, "The reason our patient experience isn't good is because we don't have private rooms." So the organization would spend millions of dollars to create private rooms. Of course, this was good for improving infection rates and good for many other things, but it didn't automatically move patient experience by itself. We'd still have to deal with other patient experience issues such as: Are we responsive? Are we answering patient questions? Do patients know the side effects of medication? Do they know who's providing care? All of this is true whether the patient is in a private room or a double room.

Another example is the newness of a facility. We all want excellent facilities. Organizations may think, *We're going to build this new building, and once we do it, our patient experience and employee engagement are going to go up.* They likely will. The challenge is, the improved results won't stay up. If we have low employee engagement, it might be in part because many times other steps were not taken to help sustain the gains: training, process improvement, or supervision, for example.

A better facility may be part of the solution to improve employee engagement. If all results are great, the new building will make things better. If the results are not great, the results will get better, then go back to what they were. They key is to make sure a great culture is now in a great facility.

We've all gone to a shiny new restaurant that had decor that just knocked our socks off. At first we might not notice the meal wasn't what we expected. But after a while, we realize the decor is not near as important as the food we're eating. The restaurant owner may have rationalized that the building was the problem, but it was more than that.

It is not unusual when an organization's turnover is high to think, *It's just compensation and benefits.* Yet after compensation and benefits improve, employee turnover does not decrease to the level that is sought.

This happened to an organization with the best of intentions. They made compensation and benefits increases. Based on market research, the decision was the right one. Turnover went down but not to the levels expected. They hired a consultant to research the situation. The company contacted people who had left. What they discovered was that the number-one reason people left was relationships, mostly with their supervisor. I believe all people in supervisory roles want to do a good job. The consultant's conclusion was the organization needed to invest to a great degree in management development. It was not a will issue but a skill issue.

In one organization, it was assumed that employees in a certain department were less happy because they had lower-paid employees. It was a pretty large organization, so we were able to look at other departments that also had a lot of employees in that same pay range. Do you know what we found? Certain departments in that same pay range had employee engagement results that were much higher. The "lots of lower-paid employees" assumption was a rationalization.

We leaders have such a broad role. Part of it, of course, is giving people tools and training to be successful in coaching, but another big part is to help remove rationalizations that get in the way of where we are. The solution is usually not very far away. Usually in the same organization there are people achieving high performance.

When we were working with one organization, infections were an issue. Yet there was a unit that had very few infections. The organization was holding 90-day leadership development training, and the leader of the unit with lower infections got up on stage and shared the steps the unit was taking to reduce their infections. The facilitator of the training then said, "If anyone's got an infection rate over a certain number, we'd encourage you to go spend some time with this person to learn what they're doing." Ninety days later, I checked back and asked him how many people had called or visited him. And he didn't want to tell on his coworkers, but the truth was hardly anyone had shown up.

There are reasons why people don't show up to learn from others. They compare themselves to the other entity and they think, *Well, they're different from me. They're a skilled nursing facility and I'm on an orthopedic floor...*or, *They're outpatient and I'm inpatient...*or, *Their employees get paid more than mine.* All of these are forms of rationalization that keep us from becoming better and using better tools and techniques that can do the job. When we learn how to relate instead of compare, a whole world of solutions opens up to us.

A question I receive when speaking with healthcare administration students is "What are the most important skills a person needs?" One I mention is the ability to benchmark. It is not easy. It takes the ability to be totally open to what someone else is doing and how the tools, techniques, and methods can be transferred to one's own area. It is hard to not start to come up with why it won't work. Yet when we learn to look for similarities, not differences, we can find solutions in surprising places.

You might have heard this story from Liz Jazwiec: When we were at Holy Cross Hospital, we blamed the homeless people who were showing up in our ER for giving us bad results on the patient satisfaction survey. It took us only about 30 days for an employee to ask that key question: "How are the homeless people getting the survey to fill out, since these surveys are mailed to patients' homes?"

Hard as it is to believe, for 30 days we had felt really good that we couldn't do anything about the problem. We felt that the homeless people were mad at us for sometimes putting them back out on the streets—all the while missing the fact that they didn't get the survey to begin with!

Not only does this story show how rationalization and blame are linked, it also shows how easy it is to point the finger at others instead of taking a hard look in the mirror.

Please don't be too hard on yourself or others if you find yourself rationalizing. It happens. The good news is we can learn how to recognize the rationalization and move to solutions.

Blame Leads to Victimhood.

Two characteristics of high-performing organizations are that they don't make excuses and that one does not hear, "That's not my job!" What both have in common is that high-performing organizations try to stay away from blame.

No doubt there are huge challenges in healthcare. Over the years, I have been involved in many, many discussions about how Medicare wasn't keeping up with the cost, the number of self-pay patients we had, the amount of regulation we faced, the cost of technology, etc. All are accurate.

There's a lot of blame to go around. The challenge is that blame doesn't get us very far if anywhere at all. It might help us feel good for a little while, but it also lets us become victims. Once we become victims, we move into this mental process that convinces us there's nothing we can do about it. We feel hopeless and helpless. And that takes away from a sense of responsibility, which is what is needed.

I joke that two islands I visit more than I would like are the islands of self-pity and blame. When I find myself blaming, next comes victim-thinking. There are certain things I can't change, and certain things I can change. It's up to me to figure out "What *can* I do?"

Often there are certain internal departments that consistently get blamed. One department that gets blamed a lot is human resources. How many times have you heard someone state, "HR won't let you fire anybody around here"? I did this when I was a new supervisor. I would just blame HR. Later, I found out that the issue isn't an HR issue at all. It was my lack of skills, which led to the lack of documentation. The problem was not human resources but me.

Finance is another entity that gets a lot of blame. I've been fortunate enough to be on some great boards over the years. And one of the boards I enjoyed tremendously was Healthcare Financial Management Association, or HFMA. What a gift it was to meet with some of the best financial minds in healthcare on a regular basis. Every finance person I've met cares deeply about patient care. Yet people tend to blame finance when things don't go their way.

I remember being in an organization that had decided not to spend money on a project. Certain leaders were blaming the CFO for this decision. One day in a conversation he said, "Well, I'm okay being the heavy." I said, "No, you don't want to be the heavy because we don't need heavies." It is important to equip each leader with the skills to explain decisions. If a leader cannot carry a difficult message without blaming, they are not a very effective leader. Leaders need the skills to deliver such news and the information to do so.

When we are blaming another party, we carry that attitude back into our unit. That's when we get a culture called "we/they." There's a good person and a bad person, a good department and a bad department. You can always tell in an organization when that dynamic exists. You'll hear people say, "Gee, I would have given this, but it got cut out of the budget," or, "Now, if it weren't for this, we'd be able to do that," or, "If it were up to me, you could, but my boss says no."

"We/they" paralyzes an organization. For years when I spoke at the Studer Group® conference Taking You and Your Organization to the Next Level, people would fill out a survey. Two of the questions were "What are you going to begin doing or do more of? What are you going to stop doing or do less of?" The number-one "stop" answer was "I'm going to stop we/they." When people realize how damaging it is, they are motivated to stop it.

Before we can defuse a we/they issue, we need to diagnose it. We can measure employee engagement to see if there is divisiveness. If there is a big gap between how employees feel about their direct supervisor versus top management, you may have a we/they culture.

Leaders can set a good example for employees by the words we use. Instead of saying, "Let me go ask administration, the supervisor, etc.," you might say, "Let me look into it and I will get back to you by _____ (give date)." The key is to be on the same page. Also, if unsure, ask your supervisor for help in messaging to the staff. That's how to connect the dots. We can also look for opportunities to manage up other departments, meaning to position them in a positive light. For instance, we can manage up finance by saying, "We are being helped by the finance department's doing such a good job of reducing our accounts receivable." Explain why that is important. Most people know why keeping infections down is important. We can help staff see how what all areas do is important.

A good step toward removing the blame barrier is to just be conscious of whether we are blaming someone—a department, an organization, an institution—for the current situation. This doesn't mean we don't recognize it. We might say, "Hey, it's really tough. The reimbursement for this has changed," or, "Whoa, there's a new competitor that doesn't have the bricks and mortar that we're carrying, so we're going to have to look at our processes to see how we can be more efficient."

We can identify external pressures. We can be more efficient. We can move into solutions. As we discussed in the rationalization section, one key is to find those who are having success and benchmark what they are doing. But it's not just up to leaders: Everyone needs to work together to find solutions. That's why it's crucial to create a culture of ownership.

How does one create a culture of ownership? There are many ways to do this. We can share the financials so employees better understand the big picture and feel a sense of urgency to come up with solutions. We can share problems and solicit their input on the solutions. We can involve employees in hiring decisions. We can ask that when they bring a problem they also bring a solution. And of course, we can connect back to the *why* behind the work people do—reminding them of the tremendous impact their contribution makes on the life of their patients.

Once people truly realize the power they have over their own lives, they will no longer feel the need to blame. You'll see a tremendous shift in employee engagement, the organization will see better results, and people in the organization will feel more confident in themselves. And everyone will feel more connected to the calling that led them to healthcare and that drives them to get better and better.

CHAPTER 5

Envy

Why did they get noticed and I didn't get noticed? Why are they on this list, and I'm not on this list? Envy is a corroding threat to human beings. It's a corroding threat to ourselves and to our organizations. Envy is a problem because it stops us from imitating success. Rather than recognizing what right looks like—and celebrating and learning from the other person or department or organization—we resent them.

Sometimes you can tell that envy is present by how people respond when you reward and recognize others. Let's say I'm speaking at a large organization. The CEO recognizes a group who has really been performing well. The CEO will say, "Let's give these people a nice round of applause." Then I will look around the room and see who is applauding. If you're in a healthy organization, everybody applauds. Most people are happy for someone else's success. If there is an envy issue, some do not join in the applause.

I was speaking at a large organization. Before I spoke, the CEO did a masterful job with his "service state of the union." He pointed out who in the room was the most successful and asked people to applaud. Well, I couldn't help but notice that some people just didn't. Here was a CEO asking employees to do a simple thing—put your hands together and clap—yet many weren't clapping.

Now, I was fortunate enough to have a good relationship with this organization. It wasn't the first time I had spoken to them. The CEO and I had a great mutual trust in each other. So after the break, I got up for my talk and said, "I have an observation. I'm looking at the amount of training that you've had. Your CEO has committed to more leadership training than most. So I don't think it's a question of access to training. When somebody is not performing well, we typically ask, 'Do they have access to training?' If they don't, then we make sure they get the training. And if they've had the training, the next question is, 'Have they had an opportunity to implement the training?' So even if people have learned a skill, if they haven't had time to practice it enough, the repetition factor won't kick in and we probably won't see the impact the organization is looking for."

Now to put this speech in context, this organization was facing the challenge of pockets of poor performance. While results were very good overall, there were still some pockets that weren't budging. Now, this organization had done significant work in leadership development training for probably four to five years. In addition, they had a great organizational training and development department. The issue was not lack of opportunity.

That day I saw a "spinach in your teeth" opportunity. I continued speaking: "We've got a challenge here: The CEO asked everyone to clap and some chose not to. Maybe people don't know how to clap. And I get that—maybe you just never learned how to clap. So you're not clapping because you don't know how. The other option is that we've got a compliance issue. Maybe you do know how to clap, but you're just not being compliant. Now this sort of scares me. If people aren't complying with a simple thing a CEO is asking you to do, like clapping, what else aren't you complying with?"

Next we did a clapping exercise. I role modeled how to hold your hands, about how far apart, and asked if anyone had a physical challenge and couldn't do that to please let us know. Then I said, "I'm going to count to three, and we're going to put our hands together. And we're going to keep clapping until I can see everyone is joining in."

Then I added, "Now sometimes we might not realize we're not clapping. So this is where, again, we need to surround ourselves with people who will tell us the truth. If you're at a table of 10 and you look around and notice someone else isn't clapping, I need you to tell your peer to clap. One way we know we have the right culture is when a coworker corrects a coworker. We have the right culture when that employee says, 'This is how we do it here. We walk visitors to where they're going; we don't point.' It's a sustainable culture when peers hold peers accountable."

Basically, we got everyone clapping and then we stopped. And I said, "Now in a few minutes, I'm going to repeat a compliment that you heard earlier about a department. I'm going to ask you to applaud and I want everyone to join in." I repeated the compliment and everyone applauded. I think in a humorous way, I pointed out a compliance issue. As the results of the event came in, the number-one comment was, "Thank you. We needed this. This is what we needed to improve." They needed somebody to confront the fact that there were issues with leaders not holding themselves and their peers accountable.

The real reason I am sharing this story here is to point out the envy in this situation. Why weren't people clapping? Of course I don't think it was that they didn't know how to clap. And I actually do think they wanted to be compliant to the CEO. I think envy got in the way. I think some people didn't want to admit that other departments were outperforming their department. Envy can be a terrible corroding influence on individuals, departments, and organizations.

Here is a personal story about my own envy. When I was a teacher, I always wanted to be named Outstanding Educator. I not only wanted it, I lobbied for it. I had people send letters to the superintendent recommending that I be named Outstanding Educator. I would never get it. The first thing I would do when I didn't get it was look at who had won it and decide why I was better than them. And of course, this was happening as I was in the depths of my alcoholism, which included victim-thinking, blame, and envy, all tied into one. One year, this fellow named John Nevins won it. And even though I liked John, I immediately thought, *I should have won that.*

Well, the next year I was working very hard on my own recovery and didn't pay any attention to the award. I didn't even know when it was going to be handed out. It just slipped my mind. I was busy doing other things, like trying to be a mature adult. And one day I received a call saying the superintendent of schools wanted to see me. I thought, *What's going on? What could I have done?* Have you ever gotten a note that your boss wants to see you and your first impulse is to start going over every possible mistake you could have made? Maybe you don't. I did.

Anyway, I went over there very, very nervous. I sat down, and the superintendent of schools said, "I just want to congratulate you. You've been named Outstanding Educator by the Janesville Jaycees." I was stunned that I had gotten the award when I wasn't even searching for the award. I was focused on my job, not the award.

I went to the banquet where they present the award. The way it worked was that the previous year's winner gave this year's recipient the award. It was John Nevins. He was gracious and wonderful, and I could see why he won the award instead of me the year before.

Looking back, I see how pivotal this episode was in my journey. Once I quit focusing on myself, my own flame of passion and purpose was strengthened. By letting myself be absorbed in my calling, I became more connected to that calling. Dan Springer, a hospital CEO as part of the Providence Health System, expressed this in terms of the paradox of losing oneself to find oneself. I thought this was a wonderful insight.

My message is to be careful about envy. It is important for individuals and organizations to celebrate other people's successes and figure out how we can learn from them.

It is up to leaders to light the way. We need to 1) be aware of our own tendency toward envy and 2) take steps to reduce it. One solution is to spend time with high-achieving people. Pay attention to what they do, and make a practice of celebrating their victories. This will help you grow in maturity, little by little. (It is human to have mixed feelings about the success of others, so don't beat yourself up for feeling envious, but we can all strive to do better.) Another solution is to focus on gratitude. When we get intentional about looking for the many gifts in our own lives, there's little bandwidth left to envy others. A happy side effect of focusing on such positives is that it helps us shift from a mindset of scarcity to one of abundance.

Speaking of an abundance mindset, there's a lot we can do to cultivate it in employees. Do as much as you can to share challenging assignments with everyone (not just a select few) and reward and recognize their successes. Offer plenty of training and encourage people to take advantage of it. Let employees know that the sky is the limit, and their growth and advancement are up to them.

The great thing about work and life is that there are always opportunities. When we lose out on one, we can assume that it wasn't the right one for us. When we keep an open, receptive mindset, we will usually find a new opportunity takes the place of the one that didn't work out. The world is a big place, and there's plenty of room for everyone to make an impact. When we model this truth, and take steps to create workplace conditions around it, we go a long way toward defeating envy and helping people work together toward aligned goals and outcomes.

CHAPTER 6

Perfectionism

Perfectionism is just part of healthcare. Healthcare people naturally want outcomes to be perfect. And in many facets of our daily lives, this makes perfect sense. Patient safety is a good example. When lives are at stake, we cannot accept any goal less than "perfect." That said, are there times when "better" is not only acceptable but an expected part of the journey to best?

The answer is yes. Sometimes perfection can get in the way of progress. When we hold ourselves to the standard of "perfect," perfection becomes a barrier.

At an administrative meeting, CEO Mark Clement was pushing for progress. We, the senior team, pushed back. We weren't ready to implement the change yet because we didn't have it perfect. He looked at us and said, "Well, if we implement it now, is it better than where we are?" We looked at him and said, "Of course." He said, "Well, let's do better; better can lead to best."

I've learned that at times we have to get into traffic. Getting into traffic means that often until something is operational, we will not know what needs to be adjusted.

I have presented at many board retreats. I've always tried to learn from other presenters. For example, a large, well-run system had brought in a consultant to assess their strategic plan and its implementation. As usual, the good want to get even better. The consultant's main conclusion was that the organization was too cautious on having to be operationally and strategically perfect. This fear of failure led to their being too slow to operationalize actions. They then explained that many times it is important to "get into traffic" to know how something works, and *then* see what adjustments need to be made.

This is a lesson we see in many areas of life. For example, my dad was a handyman and a mechanic. When he was working on a car, he would start the engine and then he'd work on tuning it. Until the engine was running, he couldn't tune it. We see the same thing with musicians; they get into action, and then they make the adjustment. Of course, they want to be "perfect," but first they work on "better."

One of our great challenges in healthcare is knowing when we need to be perfect and when it is okay to not be perfect. We can't always wait for perfect conditions before we act. One of my favorite quotes from Theodore Roosevelt is, "Do what you can, with what you have, where you are."

One Hundred Percent Perfect Isn't Always Necessary.

One of my recommendations is to outline your job and figure out what has to be 100 percent perfect, what can be 80 or 90 percent perfect, and what can be perfect sometimes, but not all the time. When we do that, we start realizing that perfectionism can do us in. Perfectionism wears an organization out.

Overcoming perfectionism is partly a time management issue. It just isn't possible to devote the same level of time and attention to everything. In some circumstances, "A" work is necessary. "A" items take time and need to be done well. Other times, "B" work is fine. It moves us on to progress. Finally, there are those times when "C" work is acceptable. There are some items that just need get done quickly and efficiently so that we move on to higher-level issues. To be a successful leader, we need to understand when each level of work is called for.

On a personal note, I have had to learn to shut up more often so that my own perfectionism won't negatively impact others. (I'm one who speaks too frequently because my mouth tends to move before my brain!)

Here is an example of when perfect was not needed, and I messed up. I was a senior executive at Holy Cross Hospital. One area I was responsible for was opening new doctor's offices. This provided better access for patients and built market share for the hospital. While I oversaw this area, there was a very capable day-to-day operator named Bill Seliga. After months of work, Bill and his team were excited to be opening one of the offices in the Beverly neighborhood.

When I arrived on opening day, I noticed that the "Grand Opening" banner was slightly lower on one end. I walked in, and they were all excited, at least until I spoke. I said, "I don't know if you noticed this, but the banner is crooked." What a dumb thing to say, "I don't know if you noticed this…" Well, of course they didn't notice it. If they had noticed it, they would have fixed it. They were exhausted, and I started off with what was wrong. I could see their enthusiasm drain out of their bodies. They were thinking, *We have worked for months to make this happen. During the last week, we worked all hours to open, and the first thing he notices is the banner is crooked!* Their faces were so obvious that even I got it.

What I had to learn was to not point out what wasn't perfect. Later on, I could say, "Hey, tell me what you thought of the event," and see if they caught it. I needed to learn not to think everything has to be perfect, because it doesn't. That banner being a little bit crooked was okay. Now, if a medication was wrong, that's not okay. If I'm not careful, that need to be perfect and point out what's wrong sucks the life out of an organization.

The key is to pause, then when the time is right, ask for others' assessment. Ironically, often the group is harder on themselves than you would be. This provides the opportunity to be even more positive. We move into the build-them-up mode.

This is one of the things Stephen Covey talks about in the great book *The 7 Habits of Highly Effective People*: building people's emotional bank account by making "positive" deposits that build strong, trusting relationships. He talks about how imperative this is. In this book when I talk about tools and tactics like rounding and thank-you notes, this is what I really mean: building that emotional bank account. When I pointed out that crooked sign, what I was doing was taking a large withdrawal out of the staff's emotional bank account.

In healthcare, people start off on a high. Molly O'Donovan, the daughter of a friend of mine, went to nursing school. When she got her first job in a hospital, her emotional bank account couldn't have been any higher.

When a person like Molly gets their first job in healthcare, whether it's in nursing, food services, security, etc., they walk in with a full emotional bank account. Our goal is to not reduce it and hopefully to keep it somewhere close to being full. There will be times when perfection is necessary, and we will need to point out things that can be better. But remember, it takes three compliments for each criticism for somebody to feel good about another human being. So we have to really load up on the deposits to balance out those times we have to make a withdrawal.

The good news is we can learn to overcome our tendency to wear people out with our perfectionism.

Looking back, I could have walked into the Beverly clinic and gone through all the positives. This would have made all the difference.

It helps to leave the subject of what could be better for another time. The owner, Jim Pohlad, and the president, Dave St. Peter, of the Minnesota Twins visited Pensacola. The visit started with a tour of the Blue Wahoos Stadium. It was in the best shape ever, even better than I recall it being in for the opening game in 2012. There were some areas that astounded me. They were white-glove clean. A reaction I had (which thankfully I resisted) was to say, "Things look great. It shows what the stadium can look like, so now there are no excuses. Let's keep it this way!" How's that for popping the positive balloon? Instead, I have focused thus far on complimenting the staff on how great the stadium looked, both face-to-face and in email.

Before offering your suggestions on what can be better, ask the staff to do so. In my case, the next time I am with the Blue Wahoos staff, I compliment them on how great the stadium looked, with a clear focus on the press box's media area and the kitchen. I ask them to take time to share what actions they took to get the stadium in great shape. The next assignment will be to create standard operating procedures to keep the stadium that way.

Also, hold up the mirror. Are you energizing people or draining and disengaging them? The best leaders energize people. Do people feel better or worse when they see you come in? What about when they see you leave? Be honest with yourself. Even if you think you are offering constructive criticism and helping people improve and be better, they will not receive the message when you deliver it in a negative way.

Finally, examine our own motives. Be careful that we aren't building ourselves up by putting others in a less-than-positive light. When we point a finger at someone, three are pointing back at us.

Yes, perfectionism is a must in many parts of healthcare. However, it is not a must in all aspects of healthcare. When we take time to identify what needs to be perfect and what does not, we make room for changes that really do improve the care we provide. We start to make real progress. Better is good. Progress is good. They both can lead to best.

CHAPTER 7

Reluctance to Seek Help

We are all human. We are all works in progress. Not one of us is perfect. And while we all know this, there is something about healthcare people that makes us reluctant to ask for help. For example, consider that one of the least-utilized benefits by those in the healthcare field is the employee assistance program (EAP). We don't seek help on issues that could really help us achieve better results.

Healthcare people are hesitant to seek help. I feel it's because healthcare people are strong, independent human beings and are also considerate. We think, *Why should I put my problems or my challenges on someone else's shoulders?* Well, you should, because you're not a bother. You're a gift.

Think of it this way: If a physician needed a medical consult, they would seek it immediately. Why not seek help for other types of issues? Whether that help is for psychological issues or organizational ones, if it would improve your well-being or the well-being of patients or coworkers, it's worth pursuing.

Also, we get better when we make a point of learning from others. This is why great organizations focus on harvesting and standardizing best practices from other parts of the organization. There are things that others do better than we do, and we owe it to ourselves, our co-workers, our organizations, and our patients to seek their help.

Sue is a nurse manager in a hospital. She is great at having tough conversations with employees, which most healthcare people find to be very difficult. Please don't think this issue is relegated to supervisors with hourly employees. It is also difficult for all in leadership ranks: CEOs, VPs, directors, and so forth. We all struggle in this area.

When somebody needs to have a tough conversation with some-one, they go talk to Sue first because she helps them. They have al-ready been to human resources to review their documentation, then Sue walks them through the best way to handle their difficult conver-sation. This matchmaking with Sue works, but if it weren't facilitated by administration, most would be reluctant to ask for her help. Why? They know Sue is busy.

Often our reluctance to seek help is due to not wanting to bother someone. We think they don't have time. I can't tell you how many people say to me, "Quint, I wanted to call you, but I know you're busy." People in healthcare know how busy they are, and they know others have a plate just as full as theirs. So they are hesitant to ask for help. We have to realize that most people, particularly in healthcare, like helping other people. It's in their DNA.

A manager can seek help from others by asking, "How do you get such great results in employee engagement?" "How do you schedule so well while I seem to be running into trouble with overtime?" "How do you hire and onboard your talent so effectively?" What I find is, it's a win-win-win: The person seeking help benefits, the person provid-ing help benefits, and the organization benefits.

This is one of the advantages of making transparency a value in your organization. It makes it easier to identify who is achieving the outcomes others want to achieve. For some it will require some ego deflation. For example, seeking help for my alcoholism was a serious ego deflation. We use the phrase in recovery "We surrender to win." This means we give up and ask for help. The win comes from utilizing that help so we can live better lives and, in turn, we can help others. This also applies to healthcare. We ask for help, we receive it, then we give what we learn to others.

In recovery, we have sponsors who help us. My sponsor, until his passing, was Norm Adams. Norm was a tremendous gift for me. Norm helped me start Studer Group®. He's the one I went to when I felt caught in a bind between staying where I was and starting my own company. I was president of Baptist Hospital, and things were going really, really well. We had great results. I had great job security and worked with great people and a great organization.

But I had this inkling of wanting to start my own company. It didn't make a lot of sense. I had a $15,000 engagement. That's it, and I was thinking of giving up a president's job for that.

Norm listened to me and told me about Emmet Fox. He suggested I read some of Emmet Fox's work about stepping out of one's comfort zone. One of the analogies Fox uses is about a father and daughter who were outside and the daughter said she was thirsty. So the father hooked a hose up to the faucet and had her hold it while she drank some water. Almost immediately, she said there was no more water. The father looked and realized her foot was on the hose. He told her, "Take your foot off the hose."

The message from Norm was that maybe I had my foot on the hose, and I needed to take it off. He walked me through the fact that I needed to listen to my heart. Norm is one of the reasons I encourage people to seek out mentors and to be mentors. Whatever our age, we can benefit from the life experience of others.

I always tried to thank Norm. And he would reply, "The one thing you and I will never agree on is who helps whom more, or who should be thanking whom."

So please, reach out for help: whether it's personal help through an EAP or it's professional help from another person in the organization or community. We all need help to achieve our desired results. When we're willing to ask for help—and to provide it when it's asked of us—our organization and the entire healthcare industry get better and better.

As my friend Dan Springer noted, when we don't seek help, we lose our potential to light another's flame and spread the calling to those we love and serve and impact—those who help us replenish our own calling…and we in turn go on to replenish it in others.

CHAPTER 8

Managing Change

While many industries must deal with change, it's probably most prevalent in healthcare. Our external environment is always shifting, and organizations must shift in response. Rules and guidelines are ever-changing. We're constantly asked to do more with less. And in the middle of all this chaos, we're expected to execute swiftly and well while never losing sight of the high-stakes nature of our work.

All of this means constant change is "normal." It never lets up. Some people manage all of this change better than others, but honestly, it is something most of us struggle with.

I was fortunate that Dr. Regina Herzlinger, professor of business administration, put me on a curriculum committee at Harvard Business School early on, where I learned so much about change management and how it impacted organizations. I was able to spend some time with people from all over the world, talking about the skills that leaders need. The normal leadership skills—communication, hiring, innovation, process improvement, supply chains, etc.—were discussed. But the one thing that came up again and again as a central leadership skill was the ability to manage change. And it is the one area where we often get the least amount of training.

Why does the ability to manage change matter so much? Because it's what allows us to get things done. If you don't know what to expect, you will often quit when things get difficult and turbulence sets in. But as we'll discuss shortly, this is exactly when it's most important to keep pushing.

When Turbulence Hits, Keep the Throttle Down.

Believe it or not, so much of what happens with change is somewhat predictable. Sometimes just knowing what to expect can be really helpful. It not only helps you plan for things, but it gives you a chance to let people know what is coming and that it's normal and expected. If you are interested in learning more about change management, John Kotter, a noted author, is an excellent resource on the topic.

So many initiatives start off well and then slowly lose effectiveness. Some call this phenomenon "sizzle to fizzle." In my experience, things start to fall apart for organizations as they hit the "performance wall." If one does not understand how to move through the wall, they may quit and begin to search for the next initiative. Another initiative may be needed, but executing on and maximizing what you started is what builds consistency in an organization.

Communication is key. Acknowledging the phases of change and letting people know what to expect throughout the process will make a huge difference. It's like when you're running a marathon and you hit the wall. If you don't know a wall exists, you're going to stop. No matter how much you've trained, if no one's ever told you about the wall, when you hit the 19- or 20-mile mark, you're going to stop. The same thing takes place in an organization.

Another analogy that comes to mind is flying in an airplane. If the pilot lets you know that turbulence is coming, when it does take place, it's not a surprise. If you are not aware turbulence is coming, it is scarier. So let people know that turbulence is part of the process. It is normal for things to get difficult at this point.

Over the years, I've helped many organizations identify and create tools to help them move through the performance wall. One of my favorite stories for helping people understand the change process is the story of General Chuck Yeager, the test pilot who first broke the sound barrier. Right before a plane breaks the sound barrier, it starts to shake. Other pilots who had attempted this would ease off the throttle when the plane started to shake, but Yeager kept the throttle down. And when he kept the throttle down, all of a sudden there was a boom, which we know now is a sonic boom. The plane then enters into a smooth flight.

The point of the story is that when turbulence hits, we need to keep the throttle down. The challenge is that people don't realize that turbulence is not always a bad thing. It means they're getting closer to breaking into the solution.

Chuck Yeager was courageous enough to challenge the status quo. He felt a calling to test the limits of flight. He was up there, and the plane was shaking like crazy, but he was still able to keep the throttle down, and by doing so, he achieved something amazing. In healthcare, we also have to be willing to challenge ourselves throughout our lifetime. Healthcare can be so consuming, we work so hard, and it can make us very vulnerable emotionally. Yet we answered the calling and we achieve amazing things daily.

There is a great scene in the movie *The Right Stuff* that shows Chuck Yeager breaking the sound barrier. If you look closely at who is in that scene, you might notice the fellow who was a little jealous of Chuck who was probably hoping it wouldn't happen. You may also notice Chuck's wife, who had a concerned look on her face and was probably wondering why he was doing this. Similarly, healthcare workers often find themselves in difficult situations, such as coming in to work every day in the middle of the COVID-19 pandemic.

Non-healthcare people are in awe of the bravery of healthcare workers, as they should be.

In healthcare, there are many times we have to keep the throttle down even though we hear messages that we need to slow down. Most of us would probably love to slow down, but sometimes in healthcare you just can't. It's not like we can go out in the street and tell people not to get in an accident, because we need to slow down.

I went through this early on as administrator of Baptist Hospital. There are three hospitals in Pensacola, and there was an insurance company that allowed their customers to go to only two of them (one of those being Baptist). One day they announced that they were going to move to covering all three hospitals. We knew right away that when they opened up access to the third hospital, it was going to negatively impact our volume and thus revenue.

I was brand new in my administrator role. I was nervous. I was probably moving too quickly in forcing changes to account for the new competitor. Some of the managers complained, and corporate brought in an organizational psychologist to interview middle managers. Then they sat down with me to tell me I had spinach in my teeth and that I needed to slow down.

At times, many in healthcare would like the option to slow down. The challenge was, I didn't have the option to slow down, just like some of you don't have the option to slow down. I said, "I can't call the insurance company and tell them not to cover services at the third hospital, and I can't call the other two hospitals to tell them to quit providing services that compete with us. I have to accept this rate cut. I don't have an option to slow down." In a way, I had to keep the throttle down.

But while I did have to keep the throttle down, there were things I could do to improve the situation. I could increase communication, increase training, and make everyone aware of what was happening and why.

In the book *The Road Less Traveled*, M. Scott Peck, MD, writes that life is difficult, and once we accept that it's difficult, it's not as difficult. I think Dr. Peck is trying to tell us that our expectations are inversely proportional to our serenity. I'm not suggesting people should have low expectations; I'm just encouraging them to not have unrealistic ones. If a person expects that when this project is finished, or this survey is completed, they're going to have a big empty spot in their work schedule, that is an unrealistic expectation. They're not going to have a less busy schedule. Healthcare people are hardworking people who will always have a full plate. Somehow expecting our plate to always be full helps us accept it and makes it less difficult.

It's easy to tell when people start feeling the turbulence. They start saying they need to slow down. But there are times when you have to let people know slowing down is not an option. I've told this Chuck Yeager story many times over the years, and I enjoy getting notes from people telling me that they are keeping the throttle down!

Making Change Happen: How Sequencing and Lack of Clarity Can Derail You

One of the biggest mistakes I had to quit making was trying to do too much at one time.

A healthcare system leader called me and said, "Quint, we've read everything you've ever written and we've tried to implement it. And we're not getting results. See here, we even have a list." And they did have a list of maybe 11 things that I've ever recommended that they had every nurse manager doing. Heck, some of them, I forgot I'd even recommended over the years. They were good suggestions, but I didn't mean for them to all happen at once. It's impossible!

So I said, "Here's what I would do. I would talk with each manager and ask, 'What's the one thing on the list that you can do?' Then start with that one. See if the dial turns. I think it will. Then go to the second item. You probably wouldn't have to go much further down the list. A few items done successfully are always better than many items done unsuccessfully."

Sequencing is so important. When I look at my early work, I missed the mark on how much change a person and organization can handle. One or two changes can be implemented quite well. Add a third item and it drops the chances of success down to half. The fourth item drops the chances of success to the 25th percentile, and then it gets worse. I see this in my own life. I have a fitness trainer, and if she tells me to do two things, I can successfully do them. If she throws that third thing in there, it's a whole different ballgame.

When too much comes at someone at once, we lose the ability to implement. Too often we take a firehose approach to change. We just turn on the hose and wonder why people are not drinking the water or not enjoying it. And we waste a lot of water. The key is sequencing. Find one change to make and do it well as you maintain the others.

Former UCLA Coach John Wooden said it best: "When you improve little things every day, eventually big things occur. Don't look for quick big improvement. Seek one small improvement, one day at a time. This is the only way it happens, and when it happens, it lasts."

The other issue that keeps us from making changes is lack of clarity. Chip and Dan Heath wrote in their book *Switch: How to Change Things When Change Is Hard* that 80 percent of failures are due to a lack of clarity.[1]

They also tell the story of how Don Berwick, then-CEO and president of the Institute for Healthcare Improvement, was frustrated by the number of deadly medical errors. He announced a prevention initiative, declaring that in 18 months, he wanted to save

100,000 lives. (His actual language was June 14, 2006, at 9:00 a.m.) To achieve this, he proposed six specific interventions hospitals should undertake and made it easy for them to participate. By the deadline, 122,300 lives had been saved. The Heath brothers credit his clarity and specificity for surpassing the goal. Their expression that "some is not a number and soon is not a time" is one that really reminds us to get clear on expectations.[2]

The message is: Don't just tell people what to do; tell them how to do it and put some hard timelines in place. Clarity enables engagement and drives execution. People like clear boundaries. Vagueness and uncertainty create anxiety and stress and make mistakes far more likely to happen. Most people truly want to do good work, and they like leaders who make that easy for them.

One more important point: *Lack of clarity often looks like resistance to change.* Many times we think we're being clear when we're not. What we think we said and what others actually heard can be shockingly different. People's being resistant to change may look like obstinance, but it's often a lack of clarity. They simply aren't clear on what they should be doing so it appears they aren't cooperating.

Clarity also promotes accountability, fosters teamwork, improves morale, and cuts down on workplace drama. For all of these reasons, clarity accelerates results and boosts the overall performance of your company.

This is why it's so important to standardize and hardwire processes and practices throughout our organization. It lets us create a high-reliability culture with little variance. Of course, this is critical in life-or-death environments like hospitals for safety reasons. But when we standardize leadership, it also creates consistent experiences for employees. Most people thrive in a culture of consistency and predictability. It makes it easier to for us to live up to our calling…and that's what we all strive for every day.

CHAPTER 9

Uncomfortable Conversations

We have a human tendency to avoid pain. It just makes perfect sense. We're taught it from a young child on. However, in the area of healthcare, there are times when we just can't avoid pain. In fact, sometimes the pain is necessary to achieve the desired outcome. Think of physical therapy or debriding a burn. The same is true in healthcare leadership: Some of the things we need to do to make the organization the best it can possibly be are painful.

One common area of pain avoidance is having uncomfortable conversations with employees, coworkers, and bosses. There are times when we know we may need to speak up on an issue but we don't want to step on someone's toes. Or we know we need to fire someone but worry that it will be hard to replace the person or there will be retaliation. As a result, we let things slide.

In a way, it's surprising that healthcare people struggle with tough conversations internally. After all, we are good at having incredibly hard conversations with patients and families. But in the case of patients and families, we have no choice. We just hope that we can somehow avoid the uncomfortable conversation. We'd rather put it off. We even learn to work around the person.

The problem is when we avoid tough conversations, we are choosing "comfort" over "character." Choosing character and doing the right thing is usually the harder path. Our avoidance prevents us from growing as individuals and it keeps organizations from being the best they can be. Because of the nature of our work in healthcare, in the worst-case scenario, an unwillingness to speak up and deliver a hard message could cost lives.

What we permit, we promote. When we don't speak up, we are giving permission to other employees to do things we (and probably they) know they shouldn't be doing.

Everyone in healthcare needs to be willing to push through their own discomfort and say something if they see an employee, a coworker, or even a leader doing something wrong. The way to convince yourself and others to choose character over comfort in such cases is to connect back to values. What is the *why* behind the rules?

Beth Keane (whom I introduced in Chapter 4), a gifted speaker who died in 2013 from breast cancer, once told a story that illustrated this perfectly. (As a reminder, her specialty was having uncomfortable conversations.) She said to imagine two employees are talking about a patient out in the open where other patients can hear them. We all know this should not be happening. It's a HIPAA violation, and it compromises the privacy of the patient being discussed. If you are a coworker who sees this happening, you know the right thing to do is confront the two people.

Now, if you're a leader coaching the third employee on how to handle the situation, you wouldn't teach them to say, "Hey, I don't want you to talk about patients where other patients can hear. It's a HIPAA violation." Instead, you might ask them to frame the conversation this way: "When patients hear you talking about other patients, they may think you'll also talk about them. They don't want workers gossiping about them so they become afraid to share vital medical info with us. Worst-case scenario, there's a medication interaction and someone could die."

See the difference? If you overheard the two others talking about a patient within the earshot of other patients, wouldn't you be a lot more likely to push through the discomfort and have the hard conversation when you realize lives are at stake? Absolutely. It's a lot more powerful than connecting to HIPAA. This is why it's so important for leaders to always connect back to values when coaching employees.

Beth's talk on uncomfortable conversations is a real eye-opener. If you put "Beth Keane Spinach in Your Teeth" in the search bar, you will find her talk on how and why you should be having these conversations.

Of course this is just one example of an uncomfortable conversation. Leaders, in particular, need to have many different types of tough conversations.

Getting Comfortable Having Difficult Conversations with Employees (Works with Bosses Too)

There are times when we have to give employees bad news. Maybe the external environment has caused a reduction in force, a piece of equipment that people were counting on has had to be delayed, or a facility that was going to be built now has to either be canceled or be smaller than originally thought. We often avoid giving the bad news, but honestly, it never gets any easier when we put it off. It's better to share the news as soon as possible so they don't hear it from somewhere else.

Just because something is uncomfortable, that doesn't mean it's not the right thing to do. Providing continuous feedback to employees is a great example of a hard but necessary function. Every employee deserves to know how they're doing. It gives them the chance to improve. One of the saddest things I ever hear is when somebody loses their job and they are shocked they were let go. In fact, hearing "I did not know it was coming" is common. That should never, ever happen in an organization that's providing continuous feedback.

We never get comfortable having difficult conversations with employees. Many of us have so many great employees, we don't have to have them that often. But when we do, it's awfully hard. It's perfectly normal to shy away from something that's uncomfortable. But remember, good, continuous feedback benefits all employees. We are never going to be comfortable with discharging an employee. If we are, we probably shouldn't be in healthcare, because healthcare people are so caring. However, we have to create a good place to work for all employees, and sometimes letting an employee go is best for everyone. We become more comfortable the more we do something. The more we can connect it to values, the easier it gets to have the conversation.

Some Tips to Make Hard Conversations a Little Easier

Leaders don't always get a lot of training on holding tough conversations. Therefore, when you need to tell an employee or anyone else that they have "spinach in their teeth" (as Beth Keane would say), you may feel at a loss. You want to say what needs to be said without damaging the relationship.

Over the years, I've learned a lot about how to hold what some call "cup of coffee" conversations. I first learned about cup of coffee conversations from Gerald Hickson, MD, at Vanderbilt University Medical Center. This is an informal coaching conversation model that's perfect for times when you see an employee doing something that goes against the organization's standards (such as Beth's example earlier in this chapter).

The idea is to say what needs to be said without damaging the relationship.

Start by holding up the mirror. Ask yourself, *Could I be contributing to this issue?* When we make an effort to become more self-aware, we may start to see a situation differently.

Speak for yourself. Don't take on the role of spokesperson for your entire team. This is a one-on-one conversation. Bringing up others throws them under the bus.

Go in with an open mind and a sensitive demeanor. You're diagnosing, not condemning. You may not know all the variables causing the person to do the things they're doing. Often, we hear something totally unexpected that shifts our perspective. You can always be wrong! Knowing this and being willing to admit it is the sign that you're a strong leader. Also, remember that the tough year we've just lived through has caused many people to be depressed, anxious, and maybe even struggling with financial issues or grief. Be sensitive and empathetic.

Stay focused on preserving the relationship. It *is* possible to convey difficult messages while still treating the person with dignity, respect, and empathy. This conversation is just one moment in time. If you damage the relationship, you shut down future opportunities for collaboration and innovation. Keeping this in mind should help you stay civil, focused, and sensitive to how you say what needs saying. In fact, tell the person up front that the relationship is important to you.

Start with the positive. As we talk about elsewhere in this book, leaders need to make three positive statements for every one negative statement. Start out by building them up before you raise the issue. Recognize something good the person has done and say thank you. Then you can approach them in a "consulting" way rather than a scolding way. This will make them less likely to become defensive.

Ask for permission to give feedback. Say, "I care about you. Can I give you some feedback?" or, "I know you are not aware of this but…(plug in the issue in a constructive manner)."

REMEMBER, when describing the issue, connect back to values. It is this connection that will make most people willing to change their behavior. Healthcare people are extremely values-driven.

Seek to be collaborative, not authoritarian. You want the other person to work with you to make things better. Outcomes are so much better when the person feels a sense of ownership for the solution. Ask positive questions such as, "How are you feeling about our partnership?" "What factors do you think led to this issue?" "Do you have any ideas on what both of us might do differently moving forward?"

When you ask questions, give the person time to gather their thoughts. Don't just talk to assert your point of view or fill up silence. This comes across as you steamrolling over the other person. This is especially important when you're dealing with an introvert who needs time to think before they speak.

Listen actively. It's all too easy to spend your time calculating your response and not really listening. Try to stay focused on understanding what the person is saying, both verbally and non-verbally. Summarize what they are saying, and confirm that what you think they said is actually what they meant. When people don't feel heard or listened to, it's upsetting. It damages relationships.

Don't exhibit a "my way or the highway" attitude. Even when you are a leader, it's good to listen to the other person's perspective and to compromise when you can. It shows the person you respect and value them. Might doesn't always mean right, and the loudest voice shouldn't always win.

NEVER yell, insult, threaten, or bully the person. This should go without saying, but we're all human and emotions can get out of control. If things start to escalate, end the meeting and reschedule when you're both calmer. A single episode of bad behavior can tear down a relationship that took years to build. The person may appear to comply in the future, but there will be an underlying resentment that affects performance and outcomes. The issue will get lost, and the focus will be on your bad behavior.

End with an action item. Ideally, you and the person will both have a task to do going forward. This way you can schedule a follow-up conversation to see if things have changed for the better.

What If Things Don't Improve After the Conversation?

Generally, this conversation will resolve the issue. The person will change their behavior. But there will be other times when things don't change. When this happens, you need to move to a "Support-Coach-Support" conversation model.

Again, start with positives! Tell the person how valuable they are to the team or how you have valued their expertise in a particular area. Then you can cushion in the "but things have to change" thought. Explain again what they are doing or saying that goes against organizational values. End with additional support like, "I know you are a good employee and want to change this behavior. I believe you will be successful. I am grateful that you were willing to have this conversation. I know it will make our relationship stronger."

Finally, if things still don't change, you will need to move to a DESC conversation, which was developed by Sharon and Gordon Bower and is explained in their book, *Asserting Yourself*.[1] DESC stands for:

Describe. Describe the behavior/situation as completely and objectively as possible.

Express. Express your feelings or thoughts about the behavior/ situation. Try phrasing your statements using "I" and not "you." Beginning sentences with "you" often puts people on the defensive, which means they won't listen to you. "I felt overwhelmed, exhausted, and frustrated."

Specify. Specify what behavior/outcome you would prefer to happen. Explain what right looks like. Use examples if you can.

Consequences. Specify the consequences if this happens (both positive and negative). Be very clear here.

The Big Convincer: Connecting Leaders Back to Values

Sometimes, even when leaders understand how to have difficult conversations, they are still reluctant. Discomfort is a powerful force. (That's why it's singled out in this book as a major barrier!) Yet I find that when we show leaders that they are not living up to their values, they are willing to push through.

Here is a technique I recommend: First I ask the person to rate how well they live their values at work on a scale of 1-10, with 10 being they walk the talk with the mission, values, and standards of behavior. The average score is an 8.

I then ask the same person to rate their skill in having performance management discussions with underperforming staff on the same 10-point scale. A 10 means they quickly provide feedback to the person on why their performance is not meeting expectations, outline support to help them, and go over the timeline during which they need to meet expectations and what will happen if they don't. A 1 means they have long-term poor performing employees. The average rating is a 5. A person usually rates themselves 3 points lower in performance management skills than values.

Then ask the leader to lower their value rating to the same place as their performance management rating. Because people in healthcare are so values-driven, this creates discomfort. Why the discomfort? The leader realizes that until they address the employees who are not meeting expectations, they are not living the values in the eyes of those employees who are meeting expectations. This discomfort will motivate a person to have those difficult conversations.

Finally, I find when people realize that delivering a tough message really *will* make a difference, they are more willing to push through their discomfort and do it. So often we underestimate the impact our action will have. A person may think, *Who am I?* or, *What difference can I make?* The answer is plenty. How would life be different if people had chosen not to act? Rosa Parks decided not to move to the back of a bus, and it made a difference.

And for every person we are aware of, there are hundreds of thousands of people who in their daily lives make a difference. Remember the story in Chapter 1 about the parking lot attendant who approached the distraught couple with the sick child and told them he was praying for them? His actions had a huge impact. I am sure it was not easy for the parking lot attendant to go up to a family obviously in pain. He could have rationalized he did not want to interfere. It took courage.

If not you, who? If not now, when? Taking the road of character-building over comfort-seeking is not easy. Many will choose not to. Be the person who chooses to act. That way you will not have to regret that you did not act. Those who choose comfort will often end up uncomfortable for they will realize they could have made a difference. When we answer the calling, we have a human responsibility to make a difference every chance we get.

CHAPTER 10

Permitting Unproductive Communication

Have you ever heard someone say, "Everyone is unhappy"? Most of us hear statements like this from time to time, but these kinds of generalities may not hold up under scrutiny. One time someone in an organization said to me, "Everyone is unhappy!" My reply was, "Now, I know that's not true because everyone has never agreed on anything!"

I was using humor to make a serious point: Don't overreact to generalities.

Maybe you have heard an employee say, "Morale is terrible here. It has never been worse." Or, "All of the employees are feeling left out!" Or, "Everyone is overwhelmed!" Now the person may be right in terms of how *they* feel. However, it would be better for them to say, "This is my opinion," rather than making a global statement. At times like this, a person may believe they are correct and/or that others agree with them because their statement goes unchallenged.

It is important to not let generalities go without asking for some clarification. Otherwise, the generality may be seen as absolute truth. What's more, when we accept generalities as the truth, we may misdiagnose the problem. This can lead us to overcorrect or underreact or even apply the wrong corrective measure altogether.

After a talk about creating a great culture, I met with an executive team. They said, "Quint, we understand what we're trying to do here is to create a great organization, but the challenge is our medical staff." I said, "How many physicians do you have on the medical staff?" And they said, "A little over 300 are our main physicians in our organization." I said, "How many of them do you feel are causing issues?" I watched them go around the room and discuss the question. When they were done, the answer was probably somewhere between five and eight.

So we had started out with over 300 physicians who were allegedly causing issues—the entire medical staff—and at the end of the process, we were down to five to eight! That's a big difference. My next question was, "What do you do with the 300+ who are *not* causing any difficulty?" And they looked at me as if to say, "Not as much as we need to." Thanking all those who are supportive is critical.

If we had let the generality drive our meeting, we would have focused our "solution" on a problem that wasn't as big a problem as first thought. Instead, we were able to walk out with a plan to recognize and really thank the 300+ physicians who were not causing issues. We also had a strategy for the five to eight who were—but as you can see, that was a very small number.

It is good to ask for specifics! By asking *how many, when, where,* and *what,* we can gain clarity and find that the solution isn't as complex or difficult as it may have seemed at first.

Often people use words like "a lot" to describe something. How many is a lot? I find the number can range from two on up. The issue is when we don't define specifics, we can end up underreacting or overreacting. We could create an even bigger issue, generating more worry and putting more energy into a situation than necessary. By drilling into specifics, we can better understand the situation, take better actions, and at the minimum, feel good that we did not support statements that we feel are not correct via our silence.

What to Do When You Hear Generalities

First, pause and decide whether you want to respond or not. There are times when it is best to let it go. Don't rationalize that it is not worth responding just because it's uncomfortable to speak up, or because you feel that speaking up may have an adverse impact on others. Sometimes you need to respond anyway. However, there are times when responding is not worth the time or the trouble, and of course there are times when a response is called for.

If you do choose to respond, start out by asking the person to explain. First, seek to understand. Using the phrase "help me understand" is a good starting point.

Next, offer to get the facts, or if you have them already, provide them. While the person may not agree, at least you provided objective data.

Don't be afraid to ask the person to provide more information they might have to support their own opinion. Yes, it is fine for the person to have their own opinion, but ask for some facts.

Finally, accept that you may be wrong. When you ask for data and the person provides it, be willing to be corrected. Be as open to the person's input as you want them to be to yours.

Carry Your Own Messages.

I have found that when we hear generalities, it's often from someone who is carrying a message for others. A manager came up to me early on when I started at Baptist and he said, "All the managers are overwhelmed." And I said, "Are you a representative of the managers?" He said, "No." I said, "Okay, why did they go to you?" He said, "Well, that's because I'm the informal leader."

And I said, "I need your help. Coach me so they can come directly to me, because I think if they come to you, it's not healthy for the organization, and it puts a lot of pressure on you to be the informal manager, leader, and representative. And I know you want this organization to be good and you want to help the managers, so I need to ask you to tell them that they need to carry their own message."

Allowing people to carry messages for others impedes an organization from high performance. It shows that people are choosing comfort over character. This is middle school behavior. Mature organizations are made up of those who are willing to "own" their views and opinions.

Plus, when people feel it necessary to elect a spokesperson, it may be a sign that you need to hold up the mirror. Is there something about the way you lead that makes you seem unapproachable. Do people feel psychologically safe enough to come directly to you? You might even ask, "What can I do so that people come to me versus you?"

What we permit, we promote. When we accept generalities and secondhand messages, we may be sabotaging our organization. We are also not doing our people any favors. We have a human responsibility to push for the facts and to challenge people (including ourselves) to get better—even if it makes us uncomfortable in the moment. Often it will be worth it in the long run.

SECTION 3

The Replenishers

You have read about some barriers that block us from being as helpful and useful as we want to be. It can be tough to focus on things that hold us back. Yet the flip side of every challenge is opportunity. With each barrier we knock down, we free ourselves up to grow. That growth is what Section 3 of this book is about: helping you, your employees, and your organization get better and better.

The replenishers are just what they sound like. They are mind shifts, tools, techniques, and best practices that help all of us in healthcare renew that sense of passion that can get temporarily depleted. They take the good work we're already doing to an even higher level. They help us get better outcomes, build stronger relationships, and keep our emotional bank accounts (and those of our employees) full. They help us get better results faster.

They are changes and tweaks to things you are already doing. They are new ways of framing familiar ideas and tactics. They are words that help others suddenly "get" what you've been trying to teach. All of this is about creating a culture in which our natural tendency to be helpful and useful can flourish, as that's really where the magic happens.

We were all born with the calling inside us. These replenishers are the embers that nurture it and keep it alive. They are also the rocket fuel that will help your organization achieve greater and greater performance.

My hope is that these replenishers will be helpful and useful as you continue your work of being helpful and useful to those you serve.

CHAPTER 11

Understanding the Phases of Learning

"People wish to be settled; only as far as they are unsettled is there any hope for them."
—Ralph Waldo Emerson

When I was president of a hospital, a new nurse came up to me and told me she was going to quit. I asked her why. She said, "I'm not going to make it." I was totally surprised, as things seemed to be going really well. My perception was that of course she was going to make it. She had been progressing nicely and was about to break through on so many things.

But then I realized: She has no idea how close she is to getting to the next level! She had begun to enter the second phase of competency and change, which is "consciously incompetent." She had suddenly realized all she didn't know and it was overwhelming. She was going to make it, but she had just gotten scared.

Over the years, I have learned there are four phases of development. We also call them four phases of competency and change. They are:

Unconsciously Incompetent: "I don't know what I don't know."

Consciously Incompetent: "I've suddenly realized what I don't know…and it's scary!"

Consciously Competent: "I'm getting pretty good at this job, though I may still need reminders or checklists."

Unconsciously Competent: "I could do this job in my sleep!"[1]

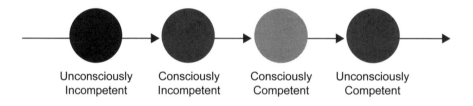

| Unconsciously Incompetent | Consciously Incompetent | Consciously Competent | Unconsciously Competent |

It is important that leaders understand these phases for several reasons. It allows us to onboard people in a way that keeps them from getting scared and quitting early on. It helps us provide the skill-building and support people need throughout their journey. This is a big part of improving engagement and reducing turnover. Finally, it helps us manage resistance to change and productively move people through that uncomfortable "unsettled" feeling.

Remember when we talked about hitting the performance wall in Chapter 8 on managing change? Learning your way around a new job or mastering a new skill is a lot like running a marathon. If you know ahead of time that when you get to mile 19 or 20, you're going to hit the wall, you'll be prepared. Because you know what to expect, you can push through it.

This is why leaders need to talk to employees (not just new ones but all employees) about the phases of change and competency. When people know what to expect, it will keep them engaged and prevent them from giving up right before they are about to break through.

Now, let's walk through the phases of competency and change one at a time:

How We Learn: The Four Phases of Competency and Change

Phase 1: Unconsciously Incompetent

In this phase, we don't know what we don't know. Being unconsciously incompetent can actually be a fun and exciting time in a person's career.

When I talk to people after they get a job in healthcare, I always ask them, "Whom did you tell?" The answer I usually get is "Everybody!" It's really neat to see their excitement. If they just got a new job in a management or supervisory role, I ask them if they went shopping for new clothes.

If you want to see enthusiastic physicians, go to a white lab coat ceremony when they're officially given their white lab coat. Their family and friends are there, and it's very exciting. The same goes for nurses: If you want to see excited nurses, go to any pinning ceremony. They worked so hard and now they get their pin. I'm sure that's how it is for almost all of the professions in healthcare. When people first start working in healthcare, they have a full emotional bank account.

But it's also a time when they probably know less about what they're doing than they will at any other point in their career. We call it being unconsciously incompetent. It isn't that they're incompetent in all aspects, but they're incompetent in knowing exactly what the job is going to be like. They don't know what they need to learn yet, because they're brand new. Though they may have an idea of what to expect, they don't know for sure.

I don't know if any of you have ever felt like this, but I'm pretty nervous with new things. When I went from Wisconsin to Chicago, I sat there and looked at the phone and realized I didn't even know how the phone system worked. At times I wanted to run back to my old job…and looking back, it was when I started feeling this way that I was moving into the next phase.

Let me add here that these phases are not always clearly divided. We move from one phase to the other gradually so it can be impossible to tell when one ends and the other begins. One thing I do know is that Phase 1 lasts a very brief time. The "new" quickly wears off and things start to get a little scary. Before we know it, we are in Phase 2.

Phase 2: Consciously Incompetent

It is in this phase that we start to realize there is a gap between our current skill set and where we need to be to become successful. This is when anxiety starts to ramp up. We realize, "Oh my gosh, now I know what I don't know." And it is scary.

Leaders have to be really careful when employees are in this phase as this is when people are most likely to quit. A significant number of people who quit their job in healthcare leave in the first 90 days. Another good percentage leave in the first year. Why? It's not that they were not enthusiastic. It's not that they probably won't be able to do the job. They get scared. They get scared because all of a sudden they are wondering, *Am I going to make it?*

I remember the first time I sat in the C-suite with other vice presidents. I was thinking, *Will I ever match up to them?*

If we're early on in our job and we don't know this anxiety is normal, we can sometimes run. I've created a seven-minute video for all employees of what it's like when you're brand new, because I don't want them to get scared and quit. We always need to provide support to employees, but we need to be especially focused on doing so during the first 90 days to the first year—because this is the time frame when people are most vulnerable.

When people are in Phase 1 or 2 (remember, we can't always pinpoint when they make the transition), that's the period when leaders need to focus on reducing anxiety. A good onboarding process can help. That's the best time to give them a partner, a buddy, a preceptor—someone they can talk to when they're feeling anxious or worried about making it in their new job.

Make sure the mentor takes the time to explain things and acknowledges that it's hard. If they have been doing the job for a long time, they may just fly through it and make it look easy. This may discourage the new employee from asking questions or make them feel they will never figure things out. One of the mistakes I made early on in an organization was assigning mentors and preceptors, but not providing them the development opportunities to learn how to be a good mentor or preceptor.

I remember years ago we got a new TV system at home and my son seemed to be the only one who knew how to operate it. I'd ask him, "Can you show me how to do this?" He'd quickly hit a bunch of buttons, give me the remote, and walk away. Since he didn't talk me through which buttons to press, I had no more idea how to work it, and continued to feel like I would never get the hang of it. So the key is to also train the mentors on how to make sure they can reduce new employees' anxiety.

Make sure the mentor knows to tell the new employee how hard the job was for them in the beginning and have them explain the difficulty they faced. During this phase, let the new hire know it's all about repetition. The more they do the job, the better they will get.

Make sure the mentor is narrating that. If you don't explain it, the new employee feels frustrated and inadequate.

When I was in college, I desperately needed a summer job. I had a wife and two kids to provide for in addition to my college tuition, so I got a job at the Ford Motor Company, racking body parts. I was afraid to ask too many questions about my pay, but basically I was paid minimum wage until I reached a certain number of racks, and then I would be paid by the piece.

I was working the graveyard shift, so I was working alone. They showed me how to put the bumpers on the racks before my first shift and then left me to it. I really worked hard. The metal would go right through my gloves and cut my fingers. The chemicals could cause skin reactions. I remember getting my first paycheck, and it was minimum wage. I had done 30 racks an hour, which I thought was quite remarkable. I asked somebody, "How many racks do I need to do before I can start getting paid for piecemeal work so I can make more money?" They said, "It's 50 racks an hour."

I went home devastated, crying, because I had a family to feed and I would never, ever make 50. Looking back, it was good that I couldn't quit. I had to gut it out. Do you know, by the end of that summer, I was making 50 and more quite easily? Why? Repetition. So the key from Phase 1 to Phase 2 of development is reducing anxiety and providing repetition of tasks.

(As a sidenote, this is one of the reasons most leaders will never be good at firing people. We get good at things we do a lot, and chances are we aren't going to do a lot of firing. There are just some things that will always be difficult.)

So as we move into Phase 3, we find ourselves getting better and better. It's all about learning and repetition. We are gaining more experience, getting to know our coworkers, getting to know how systems work. Things are getting a little easier, and we are feeling more confident.

Phase 3: Consciously Competent

In this phase, the skill set is there, but reminders or checklists are still needed to fully execute. People are likely still unsettled, but they understand the need for change and have embraced it—or at least have accepted it.

So the goal for leaders is to get people to the point where they know the needed skill. Get intentional about providing them with training and development, mentoring, and precepting opportunities. You are showing them what right looks like and giving them the chance to perform the skill frequently enough that they become consciously competent in it.

When leaders are going through this phase of change, it may help to reach outside the organization. It can be very powerful to connect your leaders with leaders at other organizations that have achieved high performance.

Phase 4: Unconsciously Competent

In this phase, we no longer have to think about what we are doing. We have reached the mastery level.

We reach this phase because of repetition. In Malcolm Gladwell's book *Outliers*, he writes about the 10,000-hour rule. Essentially, he says that's how many hours of practice it takes to achieve greatness in a skill. While there have been articles debunking this number, I feel confident that the central point—that lots of practice makes the difference between mediocre and great results—still stands.

We see it all the time in healthcare: Really skilled physicians reach mastery level because they have done the same surgery so many times.

I live in a community that has the Andrews Institute for Ortho-paedics & Sports Medicine, led by orthopedic surgeon James Andrews, one of the big names in healthcare. If you look at most sports on TV, there's probably somebody playing who has seen Dr. James Andrews to come back from an injury. He has achieved mastery.

As you would imagine, having the experience of a mastery-level physician is very comforting to patients. My father had a bad back. He had spinal stenosis and was in constant pain. He was bent over and could barely walk. This pain led to depression in my father. He also had chronic heart failure. He was scheduled to have an operation on his back, but because of his chronic heart failure, they were afraid to do the surgery.

I was very fortunate at the time to be working with the Cleveland Clinic. I was having dinner with Dr. Floyd Loop, then CEO, a great man. I mentioned to him that my dad's operation had been canceled and how depressed my father was.

Dr. Loop asked me a number of questions and then said, "Let us take a look at your father." It ended up that Dr. Iain Kalfas operated on my father's back. When he went into surgery, Dr. James Young, one of their cardiologists, was there as well in case there were any problems with his heart. Before the surgery, my dad was rather nervous. He asked Dr. Kalfas, "Have you ever done this procedure before?" Dr. Kalfas, not bragging whatsoever, said, "I have probably done more of this procedure than almost anyone in the world." Talk about a patient having confidence in their medical team. My father was excited about having two of the best physicians in the world with him.

We were fortunate to get into the Cleveland Clinic with my dad. After Dr. Kalfas performed the surgery, my father woke up pretty much pain-free. That doesn't happen for everyone, but it happened for him. Dr. Kalfas inspired confidence in my dad when he said he's done more of this procedure than almost anyone in the world.

That is the mastery level we've been talking about. Now, if this is where it ended, life would be good. You get a new job. You learn what you don't know because you don't know it. You start working on what you don't know. Now you know it. You keep doing it over and over again. You relax a little and you become a master at what you're doing. In some industries, that will last. But many industries are changing so quickly that you may regularly cycle through the phases of learning because of what you need to know to keep up. This is particularly true in healthcare, where we are required to be lifelong learners, constantly honing new skill sets because of the amount of change and advancement in our industry.

Resisting Change in the Learning Process

We have learned some interesting things about change with regard to the phases of development.

We know that people naturally resist change. But what often surprises people is that the more experienced and competent an employee is, the more likely they are to resist change. This includes positive change. The more leaders understand the phases of competency and change, the more they're able to move employees through the "unsettled" feeling of change.

Sometimes those who have reached mastery level or unconscious competence are the most change-resistant. This may be surprising, as many of these folks are high performers.

What we have found is they don't like the feeling of moving backward. If you change the way you do something, they're going to have to relearn it and may think, *Well, there's a new technique or a new tool, and it's going to take me longer. I'm not going to be as good at the new tool as the old tool. I'm going to feel like I'm going backward.* And nobody likes the feeling of going backward.

A friend of mine, Bubba Watson, is a professional golfer. He's won the Masters twice, but he's always looking at improving his game by trying a new club or a new approach. What he has found is that when he makes changes, it often gets worse before it gets better. It's the same in any job. You have to be willing to learn a new way of doing something and commit to sticking with it until you master the new technique. You're going to have to move through all the phases again. You have to be a very committed individual to purposely start over when it's much easier to stick with what you already know.

This same thing happens in healthcare. If we want to move forward, we might have to move backward first. Consider the electronic medical record. I hope when you read this, you don't get too angry, but I've been involved in looking at it from the beginning and it made all the sense in the world. People would be able to access patients' records from other places, so we'd quit duplicating procedures, and things would be easier for everyone. The medical record could even help us flag best practices at times, which would be wonderful. It all made great sense, and it still does.

The challenge was when the electronic medical record went into place, everybody knew it wouldn't be perfect from the beginning, but that didn't prevent the frustration. I remember a physician coming up to me and saying he had never worked harder in his life, and everything was taking him so long. What happens with change, particularly with physicians, is it's not the change they don't like; it's what the change can represent. Sometimes it means they feel like they're going backward on how long things take because they are learning a new skill.

It's really important when we're working with people to understand where they are. Are they in Phase 1, relatively new, so they don't know what they don't know? Are they in Phase 2, where they know what they don't know, and we have to make sure they're not so scared that they quit? Are there steps in place to give them the skills and the experience they need to be really good at this job?

Next, now that they're learning the skill, we need to give them enough experience so they can master it. We all know how this is. For example, the first time a nurse ever works on a patient floor, they're going to be overwhelmed quickly with the number of patients they're taking care of. I believe in staffing levels, but the more experience a nurse gets, the better they'll be able to handle the nurse-to-patient ratio. It's the same with any job, whether it's collecting copays, filing insurance, working in the IT department. Experience allows us to achieve mastery.

The challenge in healthcare is when we've reached mastery to have empathy and patience, because even those individuals who are good at something are going to emotionally struggle at first. If we don't understand they're going to get worse before they get better, we won't give them the empathy they need. We need to make sure they know we are doing everything possible to help them live up to their calling.

Here's an example of giving people the empathy they need. Going back to electronic records, there was a healthcare system that explained to their physicians, "This is going to be hard. It's going to get worse before it gets better, so we're going to be adjusting the RVUs for a certain amount of time to let you adjust." Now, is this change going to be easy for the physician? Probably not. But does hearing that make it better for the physician? Absolutely. Because they've been educated about what to expect and know you empathize with them. They know it's going to be hard, but they have a timeframe for learning the new skill and a buffer so they don't feel as rushed.

People are always going to be at different phases in different things. I might be at a mastery level in one activity, yet pretty much just learning in a second activity. If you have employees you're supervising, think about where they are, because they're all going to be a little bit different.

It may seem counterintuitive, but when we're rolling out a big change, the people we need to pay the most attention to are the most experienced ones. If they feel like they're going backward and they don't like it, they won't role model the change for everyone else. With proper education, experience, and empathy, they will be that role model. When they show the rest of the staff that even though it's harder on them and they feel like they're going backward for a while, they believe in the change, then the rest of the organization will follow suit.

Change is never easy. Sometimes it can be *very* difficult. But when we realize we are all in this thing together—we're all moving through the phases of competency and change in different areas of work and life—that realization can become a bonding experience. We are all on this journey of learning and growth together…and together we are making our organization stronger.

CHAPTER 12

Developing Tools and Techniques

As I explained earlier, my path to healthcare was an unconventional one. I consider myself extremely fortunate. At every point in my career journey, I have learned valuable lessons that shaped my approach to learning and teaching others. Nowhere was that more true than in my work as a teacher for children with special needs.

When I was majoring in this field at the University of Wisconsin-Whitewater, something really wonderful happened. Professor Marc Gold at the University of Illinois created a learning approach technique called Try Another Way. It totally changed the way we approach teaching children with special needs.

Back in those days, children with special needs—particularly those with Down syndrome or other developmental disabilities—were often institutionalized. Parents were encouraged to do this, because at the time, it was considered to be the best course of action. These were not bad parents, just parents who often didn't see any other options.

Try Another Way changed this reality. It was a systematic training approach based on a few fundamental beliefs: Everyone can learn, but we have to figure out how to teach; students with developmental disabilities have much more potential than anyone realizes; and all people with disabilities should have the opportunity to decide how to live their lives.

Dr. Gold would go into institutions and select a complex task that required multiple steps (for example, 10 steps). He would choose adults and children whom professionals thought would never be able to complete the task. Then, he would break the task down into bite-size pieces and use the words "try another way" until they got it right. The repetition and the sequencing he used turned out to be important keys to their success.

In this way, Dr. Gold showed that people are way more capable than previously thought. In 1975, Public Law 94-142, which is also called the Education for All Handicapped Children Act, passed. It guaranteed a free, appropriate public education to children with disabilities. This resulted in lots of students and adults coming out of colonies and institutions and moving back to their hometowns. Dr. Gold's Try Another Way approach became an invaluable resource for everyone working in the field.

I was teaching when that happened and realize that I was so fortunate to see this unfold. It taught me that when you want to complete complex tasks or implement something new, it's best to break the actions into bite-size pieces. It is a learning philosophy I have carried with me throughout my life and career. In a way, it has become a foundation for all my work in healthcare. When we make only one or two behavioral changes at a time, and control the sequencing in a way that doesn't overwhelm people, the chances for success are much greater.

When I look at failure of initiatives and programs inside organizations, the issue is usually not what's being attempted—it's the speed at which it's being attempted. People can acclimate to only one or two behavioral changes at a time. I understand sometimes we have no choice, but many times we do. So those early learnings as a teacher for children with special needs were extremely helpful to me.

The other place that was fertile training ground for learning was my journey with alcoholism. It's hard to imagine that alcoholism could create benefits, but it has for me. First, it created an "asking for help" mindset and it gives me empathy for other people who go through their own struggles. It taught me not to judge. It gave me an appreciation for rigor. It also gave me a "one day at a time" mindset, which is not a bad way to approach life.

Alcoholism also introduced me to the 12 steps. One time when I was getting a job, the organizational psychologist said, "You think very deliberately." I think it is a way of thinking that came from the 12 steps.

Finally (and this is important), another thing we learn in recovery is ego deflation. When we build our ego up, we need to be really careful, because it's going to be deflated. It is easier and less painful to deflate our own ego than to have somebody deflate it for us. This early ego deflation taught me to recognize, value, and promote the ideas of others. Once I made it a point to learn from others, and started making it a habit, the world opened up for me.

The Value of Messaging Backed by Data

When I got a job at Mercy Hospital in Janesville, Wisconsin, they wanted me to do an ad campaign. This was back when hospitals were starting to advertise. I brought in a company called Topin & Associates, and they said, "Well, we can't do advertising without knowing what the people in the community think about the hospital." So then they mentioned research.

Now, while the hospital had done research in many areas, we had never done consumer research. And so we hired Gallup. This was my introduction to the global analytics firm. It was pretty fascinating because at the time we were saying, "We care." What the research told us is, "The community knows you care; they just don't know if you're good."

So we changed our whole messaging approach to a three-point system. Point 1 was, "We have the skill." It's all in how you introduce yourself. Point 2 was, "We have the technology." Every picture we showed included a piece of high-tech equipment. Point 3 was, of course, "We care."

The big lesson was the great value of research. Specifically, I learned how important it is to narrate a story the right way and support it with facts. This would serve me throughout my career. The first time I spoke publicly was, I think, in 1989. There was a national marketing conference, and Gallup was presenting, and they asked me to come as a case study to show how to utilize data and research. It was the start of a long career of presenting backed by research.

Training Is an Investment, Not an Expense.

Next I went to Holy Cross Hospital in Chicago where I learned lots of new things. Holy Cross had been losing money, and, as mentioned previously, Mark Clement had come in as the CEO. He made some difficult decisions, and they went from losing money to making $75,000 in the fiscal year before I came on board. One of the first things he did was tell us he had just hired Dr. Clay Sherman who had written *Creating the New American Hospital* to come in as a consultant. He was going to provide eight days of leadership training: two days of training to be held every 90 days.

Now, I'm sitting there as the senior vice president/chief operating officer, and I'm a little concerned. I'm thinking, *Let me see, we made $75,000, and we're now committing $180,000. Wow. With our money so tight, why would we spend that much money on a consultant and on training and development?* I had never really been to a place that did that much aggressive training and development. It wasn't typically done back then. Of course, I was smart enough to know that I was brand new and Mark was the CEO, so I didn't say, "What the heck are you doing?"

So I went to my first two days of training with Clay Sherman, and I really walked in with some apprehension. I was thinking, *How can I afford two days of training?* I actually brought other work with me that I was hoping to sort of do while he was talking. And it changed my life. It was during this training that I learned what I didn't know I didn't know. I became consciously incompetent.

This doesn't mean I was totally bad at my job, but if you had asked me how good I was in selection, I would have said, "I'm pretty good. I mean, look, I'm senior vice president here and I've hired a lot of people." I feel if they asked me on a scale of 1 to 10 where I was, I would've said an 8, maybe a 9. But by the time he showed me what right looks like, I came to believe I was about a 4.

Sometime during that first two days, I saw that I was wrong in the way I viewed training. That $180,000 was not an expense at all; it was an investment.

Learning Together and Practicing Together Leads to Consistency.

It was during this training session with Mark Clement that I first got an inkling of how important tools and techniques really are. I found that even though everyone in our organization had certain leadership skills, we didn't have the same tools and techniques. Well, if everyone isn't doing things the same way, we would never achieve consistent results. The tools and techniques we learned during this session allowed us to get on the same page.

I found when everyone learned the same methods together, and practiced them together, we would get better and better. Our results would get better and better also—and they'd be consistent across the entire organization.

It makes sense: In a play, the director doesn't send all the actors off on their own and then bring them together just once in a while; they practice together. The same is true with team sports. Practice doesn't just make perfect; it makes us consistent. And I watched over the years as every 90 days we got together, practiced, and got a little bit better.

The Importance of Learning from Others

Around that time, Mark asked me to head up patient experience. During my days as a teacher for children with special needs, I had learned that the first thing you do is assess the situation. In this field, the formula for helping a child was diagnose first, then treat. This was another learning I was able to carry over to my work in healthcare.

Being on the South Side of Chicago, it wasn't a long trip to South Bend, Indiana. That's where patient experience company Press Ganey was located, and I wanted to learn from them. So I went and sat down with founders Irwin Press, PhD, and Rod Ganey, PhD.

They shared with me how their questions were formulated. I learned that the survey came from research on how Medicare implementations impact patient satisfaction. They taught me that some questions are way more important than others. Then they explained on a 5-point scale that a 5 is 100, a 4 is 75, a 3 is 50, a 2 is 25, and a 1 is 0. And they said, "If everybody got a 4, it would be a raw score of 75, and that would make it the worst hospital in the country."

Press Ganey didn't have a large number of hospitals in their database, but they had enough. (This is where I learned an important principle that I've believed ever since: The learning tool doesn't have to be perfect, just better than what you have.)

What hit me was that we should not be feeling good about a 75 or a 4. Compared to other hospitals, we had a ways to go. I came back with the true understanding that the goal is moving 4s to 5s. Back then it was a matter of moving the results from being *good* to *very good.*

As I mentioned, there are certain questions that have much more power than others, so it is best to focus more on them. You don't focus on all the questions to start with; you zero-in on and focus deeply on the most important questions.

Even though I had that knowledge, I still was struggling. I was finding that improving the entire patient experience is more than that.

Benchmarking Outside the Industry

I got fortunate. I was reading the *Chicago Sun-Times* and saw an announcement that Southwest Airlines was doing a management training session at Midway Airport. Because we were close by, and were one of the local hospitals, I contacted Southwest and got lucky again. Not only did they invite me in, but I got to meet Kevin and Jackie Freiberg, the authors of *Nuts!,* a book on Southwest Airlines. This is where I first discovered the importance of benchmarking outside the healthcare industry.

In fact, they actually came out to Holy Cross Hospital and talked to me about Southwest Airlines. For example, it was there that I learned about the connection between employee engagement and the patient experience. Engaged employees create satisfied customers and vice versa. It's a virtuous cycle, and you need to have a system in place to regularly measure both parts of the equation.

Another thing I learned was how important selection of talent is. One of the running stories in healthcare is that it takes 22 minutes to hire someone and 22 years to fire someone!

I learned the importance of what I would call rounding. Essentially, you meet with employees regularly, make a personal connection by being interested, not interesting, and ask some very specific questions like "Do you have what you need to do your job today?" (See Chapter 24, "It's Better to Be Interested Than Interesting" to learn more.) That was uncomfortable, but I wanted to improve the outcomes badly enough that I was willing to start doing it.

We also looked at the data and realized that some of our hospital's departments were better than others. We decided to benchmark them. When I speak at universities today, I say it's vital to learn how to benchmark both internally and externally and figure out where you can learn from others. It's not about what you are better at than them, but about what they are better at than you. What best practices can you learn, take into your own organization, and tweak to make your own?

Later, when I got to Baptist Hospital in Pensacola, we had three intensive care areas and we had small waiting rooms in them. It was just overcrowded. Back then visiting hours and visitors were limited in ICUs. Families would sit there forever because they didn't want to miss the doctor or the nurse. In looking to help make their experience a little better, I once again went outside the healthcare industry.

I had been to McGuire's Irish Pub, which is a popular steakhouse in Pensacola. McGuire's always has long lines but a very small waiting area. If there is a wait, they give you a round object that lights up and vibrates when your table is ready. They explain to customers, "You can go to our gift shop, walk around, and when your table's ready, this device will alert you." That was very helpful because pretty soon we started using these at Baptist Hospital. Yes, we were able to use a tool that we discovered in a steakhouse!

All These Learnings Led to the Creation of Tools and Techniques.

I have a great curiosity about how other people, organizations, and industries do things. I began to take all of the things I was learning, break them into bite-size pieces, and create tools and techniques based on what I had seen elsewhere.

Due to some success in moving the patient experience at Baptist Hospital, I was invited to present at a conference. The person who introduced me called me a fire starter, somebody who keeps their own flame alive and ignites the flame in others. I got up, and for some reason, I said, "I want to be a fire starter. I want to keep my fire going and help other people with their flame."

As it turned out, tools and techniques played a big role. We knew that tools built consistency. We could teach others to use the tools, get everyone doing things the same way, replicating the success in other areas, and continuously improving them.

We became world-class noticers. We got intentional about creating a tool for everything. It was so rewarding and so much fun.

Before long, we started getting hospitals to come and benchmark us. We found that we learned so much from teaching others. Of course we were not the first to discover this! Surgeons have a mantra, "See one, do one, teach one." It's a method of teaching in which students observe a procedure, perform the procedure, then teach another trainee how to do the procedure.

One of the things we would do is say, "We will teach you this for free. The only thing you have to do is bring one of your better or best practices and share that with us." That was really neat because then it wasn›t just one organization feeling they were getting and not giving. It was a mutual sharing of what works for you, and what works for us. We learned all kinds of great ideas in areas like reward and recognition, celebration, and so on.

Doable Solves Problems.

The tools and techniques we were developing were doable. And they all started with our asking, "How can we solve this problem?" We paid attention to what others were doing, broke it apart to see what made it work, and then refined it and applied it in different scenarios. As we worked with many great organizations over the years, we kept learning different approaches and implementing them.

At Holy Cross Hospital and Baptist Hospital, we found it made a difference for a clinician to say when they would leave a room, "Is there anything more I can do for you? I have time." People used to hear that and say, "Oh, this is crazy." Let me share where that came from. At Holy Cross, it was invented by environmental service workers. They would leave a room, think all was fine, and somebody would call them and say, "Hey, there's a little dust here," or, "Could you get that curtain up there?" And they'd think, *Well, I wish I would have known that when I was there the first time.*

And so some housekeepers started saying, "Before I leave the room, is there anything I'm missing?" Of course, the patient was sitting there forever looking at the same scenery, and it wasn't surprising that they could come up with something.

The nurses felt the same way. They would leave a room, sit down, and in 10 minutes the call light would go off and the patient would say, "Can you come in here?" So the nurses also started saying, "Is there anything more I can do for you? I have time." Not only did the patient get their needs met, the words "I have time" also created a sense of comfort. They reassured patients that staff were not "too busy" to bother with a request. And the bottom line is this practice actually ended up reducing call lights.

When we started Studer Group®, it opened up the opportunity to learn from so many people and organizations. An example is 30- and 90-day meetings. I was in a hospital, and we were looking at turnover. We noticed that one manager had very little turnover. We sat down, and she told us about these 30- and 90-day meetings she was holding with new employees. We started looking at these meetings and found that if we did them a certain way, we could reduce first-year turnover by 66 percent.

We thought, *Wow, that's pretty neat!* So we picked that up from this hospital, tweaked, scaled, and implemented it in countless hospitals. Now, some organizations have added this tool as a standard operating procedure into their software systems.

Another interesting one was the pre-call. We were working with an organization that had poor outpatient satisfaction ratings. One of the questions patients were asked was "How prepared were you for your test or treatment?" Now, they had given the patient brochures, yet it seemed people just weren't as prepared as they might have been. So the organization decided they would call patients ahead of time and explain what to bring, where to park, how long the visit would take, etc. What they found was that, although they'd been doing it to improve satisfaction, they found that suddenly their no-show rate went way, way down.

I remember sitting in the boardroom of a major healthcare system when one of the departments was presenting to the rest of the executive team. The presenter said since they started doing these pre-calls to prepare the people for tests and treatment, their no-show rate had gone down by 70 percent. They also shared that based on the pre-call tool, they had gained hundreds of thousands of dollars in new revenue. They had also increased productivity.

This was all due to one manager. And the CEO said, "Let's do it throughout our whole system." It is amazing how one person can do something that changes an entire organization.

I remember at one hospital they were wondering how they were going to pay us. And I said, "Well, how many no-shows do you have?" The individual I was meeting with said, "I don't know." So he called down and had a report sent to him. We sat there and looked at all the no-shows. And I said, "I think you can reduce those by 70 percent." And then I explained what we were learning about pre-calls.

This individual walked out to the car with me afterward and said, "I can't believe I missed this." And he was so appreciative, and of course was willing to work with us. I said to him, "I never did this either. I didn't do it at Holy Cross Hospital; I didn't do it at Baptist Hospital. This is stuff I'm learning now. We're all learning."

Reducing falls was another interesting topic we learned about. Obviously we knew that falls are detrimental to patients. We knew they are costly. So we started looking into why patients fall. We were lucky enough to have Lyn Ketelsen on the staff, who had done a lot of great work in response, call lights, and falls. She had a real research background, so we enlisted her to help us study the relationship between call lights and falls.

We found out that many, many hospitals at the time had a goal to visit a patient every two hours. So we basically asked some hospitals to visit every two hours. Then we said, "How about every 90 minutes?" Then we said, "How about every 60 minutes?" And for some we decided to just wait for the call lights before visiting.

What we found out is that the magic number was one hour. If a patient got rounded on every hour, call lights went down considerably. Also, falls greatly decreased with hourly rounding. We could help a major hospital achieve $1 million in cost savings by eliminating falls, and of course move patient experience results. This is just one of those things we were able to pick up by having really smart people working for us, and by having a lab that was quite large.

But here is something else that made the difference. Everything I had learned up to that point shaped my approach. Everything was broken down into bite-size pieces and introduced in stages. Today companies have taken these tools and added technology to them as the Digital Age has advanced. The way organizations implement them has gotten more sophisticated—but at the heart of everything are the basic truths I learned from my work as a teacher for children with special needs.

Be the One. Create Tools Every Chance You Get.

I get a lot of questions, and people ask me, "How do you create tools? How do you learn? How do you handle these situations?" And I talk about the fact that we're always learning from each other. We never know when a teacher's available, but as I say elsewhere in this book, when the student is ready, the teacher will appear. We just have to be willing to be a student. When we are students, we are always on the lookout for best practices that we can turn into tools.

And by *we* I mean not just me but also *you*. I mean all of us in healthcare. We can all "be the one." We can be the one who looks for better ways to do things, the one who develops new tools, the one who shares them with others. This healthcare journey is a journey of learning. Stepping up to help others learn is a crucial part of what we've been called to do.

Learning is a lifelong journey. When people ask me what I am most proud of achieving during my time in healthcare, one of my answers is professional development. At the beginning of my career, the average manager in an organization would get only a day or two of training per year. As I learned from Clay Sherman, there is real magic in bringing leaders together for two days every three months with very specific tools and techniques to learn. I still do that today with the baseball team and the various other activities I'm involved in. That's sacred.

Once we start backing off on training, organizational outcomes are impacted. At times when we need better outcomes, we can't start backing off on the tools and techniques that are going to get us there. I hope that I've had some influence, that I've been part of the solution of encouraging so many organizations today to participate in development and training. Many people tell me about their leadership development training, or speakers call me up and say, "Quint, thank you."

I get most excited when I hear from someone that they took a tool or technique that we pioneered and made it better or they have created a new tool they want to share. I love watching these tools evolve as organizations change. I also love to watch great healthcare organizations share their best practices with each other. It is truly how we all get better.

I'm fortunate to still be around. I'm so excited to keep learning. And I'm overjoyed to be back in healthcare once again.

CHAPTER 13

Learning From Each Other and Harvesting Best Practices

Back in 2010, I read an article in *Harvard Business Review* that I've referred to many times since. The article focused on why imitation is a better business practice than innovation.[1] The author made the point that while we've been socialized to think that imitation is somehow inferior to innovation, that may not always be the case. In fact, the originator of the idea often is not able to really capture the value, but the imitators do. McDonald's, for example, imitated a system developed by White Castle. Many wildly successful businesses are "copycats," greatly outpacing the innovators that inspired them.

I've always been a fan of imitation. In healthcare, the way we imitate is by benchmarking others who are doing well—other departments, other hospitals, and sometimes even organizations in other industries. Then we work to identify the "best practices" that are helping them succeed, harvest them, and move them throughout our organization.

Imitating is not as easy as it sounds. It requires us to constantly be on the lookout for others to benchmark. It also means realizing that best practices don't always translate easily from one department or hospital to another. We usually have to modify them so they work for us.

Over the years, I've shared many tools, tactics, and ideas. People ask, "How did you learn these things?" The answer is I am fortunate to travel and learn from so many organizations. The only difference between me and others is my access to so many talented people.

There are so many smart people in healthcare. When we are trying to solve a problem or improve results, it makes a lot of sense to learn from those who have already figured it out. We are also naturally curious and always looking for better ways to do things. Seeking out and harvesting best practices from others is a lot more efficient than trying to reinvent the wheel and solve issues ourselves.

When leaders learn how to harvest and move best practices, they create organizations that consistently get great outcomes—not just in one department but in all departments, 24 hours a day and 7 days a week. Best practices are the key to consistent, sustainable performance.

Find the Best and Imitate Them.

Figuring out whom to benchmark may take a little work. Often, people don't even realize how good they are at what they do. And since they don't see how others do their job, they may not even realize they're doing anything differently! They may think, *Well, everyone does this.* They're probably not going to step up and volunteer to teach others their best practice.

The thing that probably turned my career around at Holy Cross Hospital was meeting Michelle Walsko and figuring out that we needed to learn from her. Michelle was a nurse manager on one of the units. We noticed that her results for patient experience were better than the rest of the organization. We asked Michelle, "What are you doing to get such great results?" And she'd always say, "I'm sure nothing different from anybody else." Michelle loved her coworkers so even if she had known what she was doing differently, she wouldn't have said, "I'm doing this and they're not."

We couldn't figure out why Michelle's unit had higher scores than the others in the organization by looking at the reports and interviewing Michelle. So we sent Don Dean, who worked for me at Holy Cross, Baptist, and Studer Group®, to observe Michelle. (I tell people I don't know if I could have ever been successful without Don Dean.)

Don spent four days with Michelle. I know you're probably thinking that after an hour, he'd seen it all, but Don kept observing. About the third day, Don noticed that every morning Michelle took the time to talk to every patient on the unit and always asked if there were staff members she could recognize. So Don said, "Michelle, I noticed that every morning you visit every patient." And Michelle said, "Doesn't everybody?" Well, the answer was no, but the answer after that was yes. That was one of the reasons why Holy Cross at that time became one of the leaders in the country in patient satisfaction. It was learning from each other.

The More "Niched" Your Benchmarking, the Better.

The idea is to find departments that are performing well in the areas you're looking to improve. Looking at the organization as a whole is not as useful. Every organization is better in some areas than they are in others. When we drill down to individual departments, we often find solutions that debunk common assumptions around why an organization is struggling.

We've discussed how 30- and 90-day meetings reduce new employee turnover by 66 percent. Here's how that best practice came about and a great example of how drilling down helps. We were working in a large hospital in Florida whose turnover was high. It seems there were lots of explanations for why: the location, the tourists, the military, the pay, etc. But then we found a leader at the hospital who had hardly any turnover in her department.

I asked, "Is there anything you feel you're doing that has your turnover so low?" And she said, "Oh, nothing. We do the same thing everybody else is doing." (Notice she just assumed everyone else was doing the same things.) We kept digging, and she said, "Well, I do meet with new employees on their 30th and their 90th days, and I find that has a big impact."

At the 30-day mark, the nurse would ask a new employee certain key questions around the experience they were having and how to improve it. The nurse would then apply the feedback she got from the person and make any quick fixes she could. Then at the 90-day meeting, she would circle back to the new employee and give them feedback around what had been done.

These meetings were a great relationship-builder. They happened right at a critical time in the employment cycle, when new employees are at the biggest risk of quitting. (This is when the employee is in the "consciously incompetent" phase, as we discussed in Chapter 11, and needs the most support from the leader.) The new employee would feel valued and appreciated and would be more likely to stick around. So we took this nurse's best practice, hardwired it in all departments, and found that the next year employee retention skyrocketed across the organization.

Another way to identify a best practice is to find someone who is succeeding in spite of obstacles. The people to watch are those who don't use those obstacles as an excuse for not getting better. We were out in San Diego working with a large physician group, and they had a major issue with turnover. When we asked about turnover, they immediately began to rationalize: In Southern California, things are really expensive, and people move to a less expensive place.

This was a large medical group, so we started looking at turnover by department. We even broke it down by physician. We noticed that a few physicians had very little turnover. In fact, turnover was a rare exception. We did a deep dive to figure out what those physicians were doing differently and found a couple of things.

Number one, these physicians with low turnover made the staff feel good when they came into work. Number two, they focused on staff development and teaching. Staff want to do a good job, and the doctors who had low turnover invested in developing their staff and sending them to training. They had found a great practice for overcoming the obstacle.

When Identifying a Best Practice, Break It Down into Its Smallest Parts.

Sometimes we have to get really granular on what a successful department or individual is doing differently. We need to look closely at how they're doing the little things. Going narrow is the heart of benchmarking. What we often find is a best practice we can adopt just by making very small tweaks to our current processes and procedures.

At one hospital, we were benchmarking food service, which was getting rave reviews. We started looking for what the department was doing differently. In food service, one of the complaints is often getting meals delivered on time.

At our hospital, when a patient asked, "When is lunch?" the common response would be, "The trays will be up at 11:30." When the patient heard this, they naturally thought they would receive the tray at 11:30. As you and I know, maybe one patient will get it at 11:30. For the rest, it will be later. But since the patient was told the tray would there at 11:30, when it arrived at 11:45, their perception was "my meal is late."

Rick Hennessy, the director of food services, discovered that by simply having staff communicate with patients in a slightly different way, it helped manage expectations.

He would have staff give a range: "Trays will be up at 11:30. Based on your room, you can expect to receive your tray between 11:30 and 12:00. Would you like it sooner?" Ninety-nine percent of patients would say no. However, now 11:45 is "on time." Before it was "15 minutes late." So we made this small change to how we were communicating, and it improved satisfaction.

Once we figured out that getting their food tray on time really mattered to patients, we enlisted other team members to expedite the process. When the food trays arrived on a floor, a staff member would hit a bell. Not only did food service pass out trays, but everybody who was available on the unit would assist.

This process has now been implemented in many organizations; the key is taking time to study others' success and answer the question, "Is this transferrable?" If it is, then it is possible to share.

Best Practices Aren't Always About What We Do. Often, They're About What We Say and How We Say It.

When you're looking for best practices, be aware that it's often communication strategies that move the needle. Sometimes you don't need a major overhaul in a process or procedure. In fact, you may not need to change what you're doing at all. Sometimes you just need to narrate what you're already doing and why you are doing it.

Over the years, we've found it can be highly impactful when we say things like: "I'm closing this curtain for your privacy." Or, "I'm going to wash my hands to keep you safe."

If we don't narrate why we're doing something, the patient, or the coworker, or the physician may miss what is taking place. They might even misinterpret why you're doing it. Take the "closing the curtain" example. If you just walk into the room and pull the curtain closed without saying anything, the patient might think you're being rude. Just by explaining why you're doing what you're doing, you can completely change the patient's perception. If you can explain the *what* and the *why*, it can make a really big impact.

One of the more controversial best practices we've suggested is around asking the question "Before I leave your room, is there anything more I can do for you?" There has been heavy pushback. People have looked at me like, *How did you come up with this?* I didn't. What happened was some of the nurses noticed they were being called back into rooms, and they were sort of surprised because the patient didn't say anything when they left the room earlier. The nurse was thinking, *Why didn't the patient just tell me what they needed before I left? I could've fixed it right then.* Well, sometimes, for various reasons, a patient doesn't say anything. So the nurses thought, *You know what? Before we leave a room, we're just going to say, "Is there anything more I can do for you? I have time."*

These words are a suggestion. Be flexible in your wording. The reason they added "I have time" is when they asked, "Why did you not tell me what you needed when I was here before?" the patient's answer was usually, "I know how busy you are."

People got so caught up in the wording they missed the fact that they have the freedom to ask it any way they want. Nurses noticed that many patients asked something like, "Could you move my bedside table closer?" They learned that patients often asked for the same things, so they started putting in standard operating procedures, like making sure that everything the patient would need was in reach before they left the room. They noticed call light usage went way down. They had fewer interruptions, which made the nurses' work life better.

Then housekeeping staff realized the same thing: that they would leave a room and then someone would call them back to do something. So they started saying, "Before I leave your room, is there anything you need cleaned? Anything you need addressed?" These are the types of things we can learn from others. Then they get tweaked here and there, and eventually we end up with better performance.

Sometimes the Best and Most Creative Ideas Come from Organizations with Small Budgets.

At Holy Cross, a positive change happened by accident. Some changes had been made in some parts of the hospital, and people kept getting lost. The wayfinding signs were no longer accurate, and we realized we needed new ones. So we looked into replacing them. Unfortunately, when we got the estimate, we realized it was more than we could afford. Capital funds were low at the time. We decided to postpone buying the new signage and, instead, get really aggressive about looking for people who seemed lost. We would approach people, ask them where they needed to go, and then say, "We will take you there."

People loved this and thought it was brilliant, but the truth was it came about due to budget constraints. Sometimes lack of funding leads to the most creative ideas.

Here's another example: Neosho Memorial Regional Medical Center in Chanute, Kansas, wanted to reduce the number of patient falls. CEO Dennis Franks explained that they did not have money for warning bells, so they came up with a very effective program they called "Hello, Yellow." (The name was based on the yellow brick road in Kansas made famous in *The Wizard of Oz.*) They would identify patients who were at risk of falling with a yellow blanket, wristband, and socks. That way, when somebody walked by the room and saw all the yellow, they could quickly identify fall risks. They explained the program to the patients and their families, so they would know why they had all the yellow accessories and so everyone was more aware. Their falls went down dramatically. They even had a person in town who donated money for the yellow blankets. (Technology is now used, along with the identifying blankets, but the point is that sometimes budget constraints will force you to find simple, creative solutions that work and that others can also utilize.)

I tell this story often. Later I learned a hospital in Australia had adopted the best practice of using yellow blankets to reduce falls. We never know what we can learn from not only places in our own hospital or own health system, but from organizations all across the world.

Relate; Don't Compare.

To be good at benchmarking, shift to a "relate; don't compare" mindset. Rather than looking at how another department or organization is different from us, we need to get in the habit of looking for commonalities. We can harvest best practices from other people, departments, organizations, and communities that are very different from us.

I had to reduce and/or eliminate those barriers that kept me from being a good student, and I have found others can have the same issues. All through my career, I've been able to tell when people benchmarked an organization I worked with how much they were going to learn based on the questions they asked. If they started off asking questions such as, "Do you have private rooms? How many FTEs per adjusted occupied bed? What is your payer mix? What's your ratio of leaders to staffing, span of control?" etc., it wasn't a positive sign that a lot of learning would take place that day. Those questions are fine to ask, but be careful not to fall into the trap of "here we are different." (I call this attitude *terminal uniqueness*.)

When I was at Baptist Hospital, there was a healthcare system really close by in Mobile, Alabama, that had some of the best food service results I'd ever seen, so I asked our head of food service to take some people over and benchmark their great results. These were good people with poor instructions from me. They came back and gave me a list of all the things we did better than the place they were benchmarking. And there were probably many. The problem was, looking at objective measurement of patient satisfaction, they were way better than us. After the team came back in and presented what they had learned, I thanked them for their work. I apologized for not preparing them better for the visit.

I said, "I didn't give you good instructions on the purpose of your visit. There are many things we do better than they do, but right now they are doing better in patient satisfaction. I want you to go back and dig into what they are doing in patient satisfaction. See if you can bring back a list of things you learned from them. The bigger the list the better." When they returned this time, their list was just as long. We had a lot to learn from the other organization, and instead of getting hung up on the fact that we hadn't done those things before, we focused on being grateful to have learned them so we could move forward.

When we relate instead of compare, it opens us up to look at organizations outside healthcare as well. We might find other industries have found good solutions to issues we're wrestling with. For example, we might worry that our increasing use of technology—like switching from phone call reminders to emails to reduce "no-shows"—make it harder to make a personal connection with patients. But we can see that other industries have found ways to make technology more personable.

I recently made a reservation online to take my wife out to dinner for her birthday. I got a response right away that read, "Is this a special occasion?" And I replied, "Yes, it is. It's my wife's birthday." Then they asked me my wife's name and I gave it to them. When we got to the restaurant, they gave us a menu that had "Happy birthday, Rishy!" written on it. This all happened even though I never talked to a human being when making the reservation. It turned out to be a wonderful experience, and Rishy and I felt incredibly connected and supported.

"Relate; Don't Compare" Also Applies to Skills Transfer.

Another area where it's important to relate, not compare, is skills transfer. Sometimes a leader can take the skill set they've honed in one job or environment and apply it to another job or environment. It's not always an "apples to apples" comparison, but very often there are enough similarities in the two roles for the individual to thrive in both.

For example, physicians are normally good leaders. In fact, even if they're not in an official leadership role, they're seen as leaders. Years ago, Dr. Frank Byrne, who is president emeritus of St. Mary's Hospital in Madison, Wisconsin, was at Parkview Health in Fort Wayne, Indiana, another great healthcare system. He was named president and took a trip down to Pensacola, Florida, where I was a president at the time. He was really concerned about whether he could be the president of a hospital because he didn't have a lot of hospital administration experience.

A physician has a lot of qualities that parlay into executive leadership. Number one, they're good diagnosticians, but instead of diagnosing clinical data, a president diagnoses operational data such as employee turnover (i.e., when people leave, do they leave in the first 90 days, first six months, the first year—those types of things that really help you create a better culture). They're good at creating treatment plans, but instead of a treatment plan for the patient, a president creates a treatment plan for the organization. Doctors are good at giving positive feedback. When a patient comes in and they're healthier, they've lost weight, their metrics are better, doctors are very complimentary. Doctors are also good at delivering tough messages because they must deliver them to patients. As I expected, Dr. Byrne went on to be a great leader.

Don't Wait for Proof That a New Practice Works 100 Percent of the Time.

Healthcare people are scientists. We like plenty of evidence that something works before we are willing to change our processes. But don't assume you need to wait for a validated study. If you see a best practice you suspect might work for you, try it right away.

Often in healthcare, our instincts help us see connections with cause and effect before there is adequate research to validate our instincts. Those who act on these instincts are the first movers. The work of first movers helps gather the data to either validate or invalidate the instincts that drove the action of the first movers. We used to *think* there was a correlation between employee turnover and quality, employee turnover and finance; now we *know* it.

Research shows there's a connection between employee satisfaction and patient experience, and turnover has a big impact on both metrics. Why? If an employee is new, maybe they don't have the hand-offs right yet, maybe they're not comfortable saying the right key words, and so on, and that affects the patient experience. Also, turnover is quite costly.

When we realize the huge payoff of reducing employee turnover, the value of being a first mover becomes clear. Chances are, you have nothing to lose by implementing a best practice and everything to gain. As long as it's better than what you have been doing, try it.

Often the Answer Is Within the Organization.

We often think benchmarking requires that we look outside the organization, but that's not always true. There are usually leaders inside an organization who are achieving great results. Because people don't want to brag, it is important that we get intentional about finding and learning from them.

Often it's a matter of seeking out people who are doing well in the area you want to improve and asking for feedback: "Please be honest with me…what could I do better?"

I remember visiting a hospital that started posting the ED physicians' patient experience results in the staff breakroom. A physician noticed that his results were not as good as others. In this ED, the doctors rarely worked at the same time, so observing each other was difficult. So one day he asked one of the nurses who worked with all of them, "What are some things they're doing that you notice I'm not doing?" She shared a list of small improvements he could make based on what she saw others doing, and he thanked her because he wanted to improve. From her vantage point, she got to see all of the physicians work, so she was a perfect person to harvest best practices from.

Once you realize someone inside your organization has figured out a best practice, you can often get them to train the rest of the staff. When I was the president of a hospital, the ED physicians shared that some of the nurses didn't have the needed skill set for the ED. I asked, "What skills would you like them to have? Would you, the physician group, be willing to teach the nurses the skills you want them to have? Instead of sending them somewhere else, we'll figure out how to pay you to be the instructors."

They said yes. And they did it. It hardly cost us anything, because these doctors really wanted these nurses to be successful. If the nurses were successful, that was a good indication that the doctors were good teachers. The physicians bonded with the nurses during the skill-building. They took pride in the success of the nurses.

A Few Closing Thoughts

Before we wrap up this chapter, I'd like to share a few more "best practices on best practices." One is to benchmark new employees. In other industries, employers make it a priority to harvest intellectual capital. We can do the same in healthcare.

We do this simply by talking to new employees. If you have 30-day meetings in your organization (as described earlier in this chapter), make sure one of the questions you ask is: "At your previous hospital, what are some things you saw already in place that you feel could make us better?"

By asking this early, before the new employee gets too engrained in the new system, you can catch them before they forget the best practices they already knew. You'll benefit from their fresh perspective, and they feel valued and appreciated.

In fact, David Callecod, my long-time friend and fire starter who has achieved 99th percentile results in patient/employee/physician engagement at critical access, rural, suburban, and urban hospitals throughout his career, would attend general orientations and greet all new employees. In his presentations, he would always say, "We are not silly enough to think we have all the best processes or the best ways of doing things here. So use your fresh eyes, and please, please, please, in your first 30 days with us, let us know if there was a better practice at your last hospital or place of work. Take notes and be ready to discuss it with your supervisor at your 30-day meeting. We want to always get better, and we value what you bring to this organization."

David shared that there were an amazing number of better practices introduced at his hospitals, because of this emphasis, many of them coming from outside the healthcare setting.

Also, get intentional about sharing your own best practices. Learn to notice the things you do well and make a point of sharing them across your organization and with other organizations.

Finally, take advantage of technology. Today so many great companies provide technology for almost every tool and technique I've written about in my books. This means the tools and techniques are more accessible and easier to share with others than ever before. The more we share best practices, the more consistency and sustainability we achieve. The more consistent and sustainable our organizations are, the more equipped we are to fulfill our calling and serve the patients who put their trust in us.

People sometimes ask me, "Where did you learn all these things?" The answer is, I learned them from you. I learned them from being out and about. I learned them from reading what you're doing. I learned them from paying attention when I initially visited you. I learned them from following up.

When the student is ready, the teacher appears. You have all been my teachers. And the great thing about healthcare is we're used to being students. We're called to be students. The better students we are, the more helpful we can be, and the more useful we can feel. We never stop being students. The further we go, the more we realize we don't know. The more open we are to learning from others, the better we'll be…and the more we'll have to share with those who come after us.

CHAPTER 14

Why Standard Operating Procedures Are So Powerful

Clearly documented, step-by-step procedures and checklists that are easy to follow are the foundation of a well-run organization. There are many reasons why this is so. The biggest reason is that they eliminate ambiguity around how things should be done. Not only do people appreciate the clarity (it reduces anxiety), having standard operating procedures (SOPs) in place creates the consistency and sustainability that allows your organization to thrive.

Standard operating procedures give people time, which is one of the most valuable things we have. One of my favorite books is *The E-Myth Revisited* by Michael E. Gerber. One of Gerber's main points is how important it is to work *on* your job rather than always working *in* your job. If you spend all your time working *in* your job, performing your day-to-day activities, you won't have any time to work *on* your job, making big picture improvements that will benefit your organization in the long-term. Hardwiring systems and standard operating procedures allows us to get things right the first time, which saves valuable time.

The following example is not from healthcare, but the underlying principle is the same. My wife owns a coffee shop, cafe, and olive oil store called the Bodacious Shops on the corner of Palafox and Main in Pensacola, Florida (and in Janesville, Wisconsin). People love their dogs, so putting out a water bowl on the sidewalk in front of the shop every day makes a difference. People who walk their dogs downtown really appreciate the water dish. And the people who don't have dogs also think it's a nice thing to do. The challenge was, some days the bowl was out, some days it wasn't; some days the bowl was brought in, some days it wasn't.

When we looked at the standard operating procedures for opening the shops, putting out the water bowl wasn't on the list. So that meant that somebody had to constantly be reminded to put it out in the morning or bring it in at the end of the day, or the supervisor had to do it. Filling water bowls every day would be considered working *in* your business. Working *on* your business would be adding water bowls to your SOPs so it gets done consistently without the supervisor having to remind someone to do it.

The same thing goes for our personal life: We can work *in* our life or work *on* our life. Of course, working *in* our life means that we're doing the things we need to do daily. Working *on* our life means identifying SOPs for ourselves—taking a step back to look at some changes or adjustments we can make to save time we can then spend doing the things we truly enjoy.

A Few Benefits of Creating SOPs

Here are some good reasons why we need to create SOPs inside our organization:

It helps create consistency and sustainability and helps hard-wire consistent excellence. If everyone has an agreed-upon way of doing something and that's well communicated and documented, it greatly reduces the chances of mistakes. Both employees and patients will have a consistent experience. Imagine what this will do for productivity, morale, and so forth.

It's a huge time saver. Standard operating procedures may supercharge efficiency. People will move quickly through tasks and be able to get more done.

It helps eliminate frustrations by creating predictable work environments. No doubt the work environment can and often does play a role in burnout. When we create clear expectations and a more predictable work experience, we may be able to prevent burnout, at least in some instances. Employees want consistency and predictability in their leaders and their work life. Patients too want consistency in their experience and are happier when they receive it.

It prevents Park Ranger Leadership by allowing for more workplace independence. What I call Park Ranger Leadership is the attitude that leaders will swoop in and rescue employees if they get "lost in the wilderness." We help people so much that they quit helping themselves. Good standard operating procedures prevent much of this behavior because the "how to" is clearly spelled out, and employees don't have to come to you for everything.

It's a great onboarding, training, and employee development methodology. By standardizing orientation and training procedures, new employees learn the "lay of the land" more quickly. In fact, any time an employee (new or not) needs to learn a new skill, having SOPs in place reduces the learning curve.

It helps sharpen skills for those who are struggling. By referring them to the SOPs, you can clearly show them what "right" looks like. This gives the employee a better chance for a win. It also gives leaders something to hold them accountable to.

It helps with work transfer. When a key staff member is not available for whatever reason, work does not have to come to a stand-still. By referring to the SOPs, a leader can make it easier for someone else to take over the urgent tasks.

SOPs should be created with plenty of input by employees. Make sure all steps are carefully thought-out and documented so they'll make sense in the future. (It's very easy to forget them when a little time has passed.)

Don't think of your SOPs as something to put in a binder on a shelf and rarely look at. They are living documents to revisit often and adjust as needed.

Success Plates Can Help.

A good way to start compiling your SOPs, or enhance them if you already have them, is by creating what I call "success plates." We've all heard of templates. Success plates are very similar. They're a way of immediately capturing what went well—and more importantly, *why* it went well—right after a successful event, a good day, or some other positive occurrence.

I've learned this from a number of people in healthcare. One of the first was Dr. Jay Kaplan, an emergency room physician. He shared with me that when the ER had a really good day, they would give a short survey to all the employees who worked that day to ask why they thought the day went so well. You might assume the answer would usually be "we didn't have a lot of patients," but that wasn't the case. They surveyed the staff on really busy days when things went well. The survey identified those items/actions that made for a good day. This became a success plate—a document that spelled out what need-ed to happen to create a productive day.

Dr. Kaplan pointed out that the immediacy was the key. What had happened was fresh on everyone's mind, so it was a lot easier to identify the particulars. Sometimes we might assume we know what went right, but when we really start drilling down, we discover the real success factor was something else entirely.

Success plates also allowed them to celebrate what was going well (which was important for people's morale), and to reinforce what right looked like. This in turn helped them carry the momentum of a good day over to the next day.

So, the systems were working, the staffing was right, certain physicians were working, and this really helped them discover how to hardwire certain aspects of what needed to happen during the shift to make sure that it was a successful shift. It also reminded people that today was a good day and really forced them to identify and focus on what was going well. This may not happen otherwise. In healthcare, we have the tendency to study only when things go wrong, which makes sense. When something goes wrong, we need to analyze it to figure out what went wrong and why, so we can prevent it from happening again.

My suggestion is we spend the same amount of time analyzing when things go right.

An emergency department in a large medical center in California had made some tremendous improvements, so I asked to meet with the staff. I asked them, "What are you doing now that you weren't doing before?" I find that the best time to ask those questions is when people are feeling good. If I meet with people when things aren't going well, they tend to be worried, defensive, and sometimes don't share much.

It was an interesting meeting. As soon as I asked the question, one of the staff members said, "Well, we were supposed to go out into the waiting room and update families on wait time every 20 minutes. We had quit doing that. This last month, we started it up again, and you can see it has an impact." When we have success, we need to analyze why so we can figure out what right looks like and keep doing it.

When I speak to university students, they often ask what advice I would give someone when they're looking for a job. One of the suggestions I give is to ask the interviewer this question: "If you offer me this job, and I accept it, a year from now what would I have to have accomplished for you to consider me an outstanding hire?"

Asking this question creates clarity. It helps the applicant know what right looks like and what the desired outcomes are. I believe, too, that the interviewer walks away impressed that the applicant is so results-oriented. I've seen this happen in the area of consulting. Mark Clement taught me this. When he was interviewing a consulting company, he said to them, "Tell me who is your best client you've ever worked with and exactly what they did to make them the best client so we can do the same thing if we utilize your services."

Bingo. What Mark did was help the consultant teach us what the best client did. That's an approach I've always recommended since then. It goes the other way too. The consultant can say to the organization, "Tell me the best consultant you've ever worked with, who achieved the results we all want. And tell me exactly what made them your best consultant." These are methods to capture what right looks like and will help you figure out your next steps.

It also allows us to create and hardwire standard operating procedures for success. When a project doesn't go well, we do what Jim Collins calls "an autopsy without blame" in his book *Good to Great*. In an autopsy without blame, you don't focus on who made the mistake. You focus on internal systems and processes to make sure the same mistake doesn't happen again.

Well, why not do an autopsy after a successful project? If a project exceeds expectations, step back and figure out why it went so well. A successful implementation usually has clarity around goals and time-lines, priorities are in order, employees receive training and development, and so on. Each organization should have its own standard operating procedures in place to help them implement new projects effectively.

In healthcare, we always say we want to get better and better, and we truly do want that. SOPs and success plates give us a way to actually do this. They help us put our actions where our hearts are.

CHAPTER 15

Reward, Recognition, and the Power of Thank You

We humans thrive on being appreciated. Yet the memories we visit again and again have little to do with money or grand accolades. Often it's the simple, heartfelt words and gestures of gratitude that stick with us. I've seen this truth again and again throughout my career. Never underestimate what "thank you" can mean to someone.

One hospital had a creative way of recognizing its employee of the month. After the person was chosen, a box was then placed in the cafeteria. It featured a story on why that person was named and included index cards for staff to fill out if they wanted to. Staff members would write their own thank-you, a word of congratulations, a personal story they wanted to share, etc. At the end of the month, the recognized employee would receive the collected index cards. They would also receive an employee-of-the-month pin to wear.

A manager in that same hospital told me a story that taught me not to underestimate the power of such gestures. She went to the wake of an employee who had passed away. When she walked up to the casket, she noticed that on his lapel was his employee-of-the-month pin. And in the casket were the many index cards he had received. The wife shared with her what a huge thing that was to him that as he was dying, he kept those cards by him and kept reading them.

Speaking at another organization, I asked how many of them had gotten a thank-you note from someone in the organization. This was an organization that had adopted a system to recognize people. I was amazed at how many hands went up. I said, "Just think about that. What do you do with them?" A fellow sitting on the front row asked, "Would you like to read mine?" I said, "Well, sure." He opened up his book that he carries with him to take notes at work and there on the left side was his thank-you note. When do people throw away their thank-you notes? You know the answer. The answer is never.

Many people seem to find handwritten notes to be the most meaningful. Dr. Kevin Post, CMO of Avera Medical Group, said when he learned about the power of handwritten notes it inspired him to commit to doing more of them, rather than sending emails that can be easily deleted.

It's those types of things that really make an impact on somebody. In healthcare, people work so hard. They do so many things to get recognized for: so many that at times they may feel they are being taken for granted. Letting people know we appreciate them, we care about them, and we are thinking about them is invaluable. Reward and recognition is so important. We often know such actions make a difference; however, I feel we underestimate just how much of a difference it is.

Rather than building a culture that focuses on what's wrong or what we could improve, we can build a culture of appreciation, recognition, and usefulness. Don't underestimate the impact appreciation has. It builds up that emotional bank account that's so crucial for keeping people engaged and connected to passion and purpose.

In my case, I had to quit believing a myth I had heard around positive recognition, which was that we can use it to balance out the negative. "Balancing out" is a fallacy. I have come to learn that it takes at least three positive interactions for each negative for one person to feel good about the other person. A 2-to-1 "positive-to-negative" ratio creates a neutral feeling, and a 1-to-1 ratio creates a negative feeling.

So it takes three positives for every criticism for an employee to feel good about a leader. If I just keep pulling somebody in and telling them what they're doing wrong, they're going to hear from me or even see my name and go, "Ugh." Just think about it. Many times when I speak, I say, "If you got a text right now from your boss that read, 'Call me at the next break,' is your first thought, *Oh, good. Here comes reward and recognition?* No. It's probably, *Yuck. What did I do now?*"

In fact, early in my career, an organization I worked at had a system in place based on what mood the CEO was in that day. The secretary there knew the system, and she would even say, "Now is not a good day." What's more, if she knew it was a good day, she'd actually call you and say, "Now's a good time to come and ask for something." We joked that we wished we could hang flags outside the CEO's door. A red flag would mean "don't come in." A yellow flag would mean "be cautious." A green flag would mean "it's a good time to come in."

The message here is that we want to coach in a way that helps the person hold up the mirror and addresses behavior issues. But we want to do it in a way that doesn't create a relationship where people assume every time they see us it's going to be bad news. Of course, if it's a situation where all you have is bad news and negative feedback you may need to ask, "Is this the right person to be in this role?" But most people in healthcare, probably 98 percent of them, *are* the right people for the role.

We've always known research shows the number-one thing employees look for in their boss is "Does my boss care about me as a person?" In healthcare, I think caring for a person means, "Am I doing everything I can to create the right environment for them to work in? Am I making sure that I'm developing them?" And at times, it also means recognizing the good work they do.

I share this because I have heard people rationalize not recognizing people. They might say, "I just told them they did a good job a few weeks ago!" It is like we have a limited supply of recognitions in us, and when they are gone, we have no more. The truth is the opposite: The more we recognize, the more the behaviors are repeated, and our recognition chips are always replenished. When an athlete makes a good play, or a singer belts out a great song, we don't think, *I don't need to applaud; I did it the last game or performance.* Recognized behavior gets repeated. We cannot give too much positive recognition!

Also, reward and recognition is vital for talent retention. People want to be where they feel appreciated. This is true everywhere, but it is *especially* true in healthcare.

Don't Wait for Huge Milestones or Perfect Results to Reward and Recognize.

Healthcare workers are stoic individuals. They don't do their jobs to be rewarded and/or recognized. However, it is nice when it happens. My experience is it is easy to fall into the trap of recognizing only when someone goes above and beyond. But just going to work every day in healthcare, with its ups and downs and pressure to provide great care, is worthy of being recognized.

I think it's really important to recognize and reward people where they are. That doesn't mean you're always going to reward and recognize them for that behavior. You can gradually raise the bar. For example, when I was at Holy Cross, we held a hospital-wide celebration when we hit the 40th percentile in patient satisfaction. Some might think, *How can you celebrate being in the 40th percentile?* Well, considering we had been in the single digits, getting to the 40th percentile was pretty strong. I contemplated updating my résumé to read that we had quadrupled patient satisfaction while I was there. We celebrated the progress. But then we raised the bar and said, "Now our next goal is to get to the 60th percentile, then 75th, then 90th, then 99th." Eventually we were in the top one percentile in patient experience.

We then had a month when we dropped from the high 90s to the low 80s in patient experience. That happens. It's normal to have some ups and downs. But at times we have to celebrate the milestones along the way to get to the end result.

Sometimes we hold back on celebrating along the way, because people think they don't need reward and recognition, but they do. Physicians need to be recognized as much as anyone else. I could tell story after story about physicians being recognized and what it means to them. (More on this later.)

Other industries recognize people for consistently doing their jobs. I'm a baseball person. For those of you who have ever watched baseball players, you know they get rewarded and recognized for just doing their job. Cal Ripken Jr. is one of my favorite examples. He got rewarded and recognized for perfect attendance. By perfect attendance, I mean he played in consecutive games without missing a game. In baseball, if you are injured and don't play or you're tired and need a break, you still get paid for those games.

On September 6, 1995, Cal Ripken broke Lou Gehrig's record of 2,130 consecutive games played, which many people thought would never be broken. Do you know when he broke Lou Gehrig's record, national television interrupted programming to show him breaking the record? They actually stopped the game and he ran around the entire field, even the outfield, with the fans waving and yelling and he spoke about how it felt to break the record. Cal Ripken was earning about $7 million a year back then, but they rewarded and recognized him for just doing his job.[1]

Why don't we recognize more often in healthcare? Sometimes we set the bar too high. We use words like "above and beyond." I think needing to go above and beyond is a bit of a stretch. We have to be willing to recognize people for consistently doing what they've been hired to do.

Somebody once asked me, "Do you mean we should recognize people just for coming to work?" I said, "It's not a bad idea." Behavior that gets rewarded and recognized gets repeated.

Be As Specific As You Can with the Recognition.

Sometimes I ask an organization: "How often do you recognize people?" After they answer this, my next question is "Is it group or individual recognition?" I find that recognition tends to happen more in groups. Typically this is not the ideal. A key action to eliminate or reduce is accepting generalized statements. The same goes for making generalized statements.

Of course, on some occasions, generalized statements are better. The key is to be sensitive to how often they happen. At times, we want to say that everybody's doing a good job. Certainly this is true during the COVID-19 pandemic of all healthcare providers.

Still, we need to try to make them as seldom as possible. I've learned over the years, it's not uncommon to hear, "I just want to thank everyone. You all do a great job." The challenge with that is the people who really *are* doing a great job won't think as much of it if they know people in the room who are also hearing the recognition are *not* doing a great job.

Actually, it's a double loss. The people you want to compliment aren't taking it as a compliment because they're thinking, *Well, gee, that person isn't doing a great job. In fact, they haven't even been here for the last three days.* Meanwhile the people who aren't performing well now feel they're okay, because you've just told them they do a great job. Then when the person is given less-than-positive feedback, they may say, "You just complimented me. You told us everybody in the unit was doing a good job." You can see the confusion.

I understand why we fall into this trap of general compliments, but we need to be careful not to do it too much. The best way is to always be as specific as you can. The more specific you are, the more the person will appreciate the recognition. The more specific the compliment, the more meaningful it will be.

I have shared the power of handwritten notes for many years. I learned this from my grandfather, but ironically, he didn't write handwritten notes. My grandfather had one arm. When he was in his thirties, he worked for Missouri Pacific Railroad. He fell down on an icy track and a train severed his arm. So my grandfather had to either type his letters with one hand or dictate them. So all of his letters that I've talked about making such a big impact over the years were typed. While I like handwritten notes, typed notes work too as long as they are specific—and the more specific, the better.

People sometimes ask me, "Well, Quint, can you still recognize somebody who's performing poorly?" I say, "You can, but you just want to make sure it's very specific about what they do well." You don't want to say something like, "You're an outstanding employee." What you can say is: "On this day, I noticed that you did this (and spell out the behavior). This behavior is excellent."

By the way, it's important to own recognition for those you directly supervise. As my cousin Al says, "You spot it, you got it." In other words, if you spot that those you lead need support to feel valued, then it is up to you to provide that support. Don't think you are not important enough and that it would be better for your leader to do this. This goes for public team recognition, notes written and mailed to the person's home, and other ways to say thank you and help those you lead to feel valued. Once you feel it is up to someone else to make it happen, you have shirked your role.

Look for Opportunities to Recognize Family Members.

It is not enough to say thank you only to employees. We need to recognize their families also. Healthcare work is hard, stressful, time-consuming, and emotionally demanding. The pressure often spills over to the families of physicians and employees. They end up having to make a lot of sacrifices. When we acknowledge this truth, it means a lot to our care teams and also to their family members.

In one organization I worked with, we had a situation where one of the doctors literally spent the whole weekend in the hospital due to the care some patients needed. The staff knew that the physician's partner was going to be impacted because they knew how much home responsibility there was. The next week, the staff got together and sent flowers with a note to the partner, thanking them for understanding and acknowledging that the weekend was tough on them too. That person got the flowers, read the card, came to the hospital, went up on the nursing unit, and cried and said, "I've never had anything like this happen to me."

While it may have seemed like a small gesture to the staff, the impact on the physician's partner was huge. It's so vital to thank the family members of our healthcare workers. I know many of you do this, and it doesn't go unnoticed.

Here's another example of the impact recognition can have on family members. A single mom got a nice note from her boss and put it on her mantle at home. Soon after, her tween daughter had a slumber party. When her daughter was showing the girls around the house, she stopped by the mantle and showed every one of her friends the note her mom had received from her boss. The mom saw what an impact the note had on her daughter, and it inspired her to leave her daughter a note on the mantle telling her how much she meant to her.

Here's one last story about impacting family members through recognition. In a radiology department I worked with, the staff loved the radiology manager. I wondered, *What does this person do to create such loyalty?* The manager did a lot of things, but one of the things that stood out to me was they sent a birthday card to every child of every employee. This had a huge impact on the kids and made them feel appreciated.

Ever since then, my wife and I have sent birthday cards with $25 to every employee's child who is below the age of 18. (I know this is impossible financially for many due to the number of employees you may have, but we have enjoyed doing it.) We've done this since 2000 and it has been wonderful. And we get these great thank-you notes from the children.

Now please don't think sending a birthday card to employees' children is going to make up for deficiencies in leadership. But it is an inexpensive way to let your employees know you care about them and their families, and it can have a tremendous impact on how they feel about you and the organization.

Physicians Need Appreciation, Too.

As I mentioned earlier, physicians may act like they don't need reward and recognition. This is not accurate. Every human being craves that feeling of appreciation, of knowing they make a difference, even if they may not show it.

I was talking with Dr. Elizabeth Aubry, chief of staff for the VA Long Beach Healthcare System, recently about how hard doctors work, almost always without complaint. As I listened, the incredible work these physicians do and the impact they have was again reinforced, which is all the more reason we should find ways to say thank you to these incredibly valuable individuals.

A healthcare system I worked with held big quarterly physician meetings where they recognized physicians with high patient experience results. It was a large system, and based on their location, some physicians had to travel 45 minutes to an hour to be at the quarterly events.

They had a doctor who, due to travel time and family obligations, did not attend the quarterly meetings. It happened that I was there to present and be part of the ceremony when she was on the list to be recognized. They said, "She will not be here. She's never come to one of these yet." As they were saying it, guess who walked in the door? She did. They underestimated what the recognition for something she valued meant to her.

Remember, the majority of physicians are strong I's on the Myers-Briggs Type Indicator ("I" stands for "Introvert"). That means something can be really important to them on the inside, but they might not express it as much on the outside. Being introverted, steady, and consistent can help physicians in their job because if they wore their emotions on their sleeve, it could create anxiety for their patients. However, sometimes others can misread introverts and think they're not as engaged or that they don't care as much.

Doctors appreciate reward and recognition just like everybody else. I could write a whole book on stories about this. To celebrate National Doctors' Day, a healthcare system in Boston asked all the staff to write letters about what physicians meant to them. People poured out stories about what they'd seen members of the medical staff do, including some who had their own personal healthcare experience with some of the doctors on the staff. They were extremely strong, positive stories about the impact physicians make. They then posted the letters of recognition along the hallway to the cafeteria.

What was beautiful about this was that the hallway was filled with doctors for that week, reading what had been written about them. It turned out even better than planned because visitors were reading the letters too. If your family member or friend were in the hospital, wouldn't you want to read all these great things about the doctors who work there?

The letters had such a positive impact on the doctors that for Nurses' Week, they asked the doctors to write letters about what nurses meant to them. Almost 100 percent of the physicians wrote something. Many doctors were better at sharing their appreciation in writing than verbally. (This is not unusual for introverts.) One doctor even wrote a beautiful poem expressing how important nurses are to doctors.

It was a wonderful experience for all. Just by making a point to celebrate their medical staff, this health system opened a floodgate of appreciation and positive feelings.

Finally, Recognize Leaders for All They Do.

We've talked a lot about thanking employees and thanking doctors, but we also need to take time to thank leaders. These are challenging times for many leaders. Don't be afraid to write them a note of appreciation and recognition for all they do.

There was a CEO who worked at corporate headquarters who most people in the organization never saw due to the size of the system. The president of one of the local hospitals was talking about thank-you notes and said, "I wonder if the CEO gets many notes." He said, "He's been here a long time and done a lot of great things for this organization. Some of us have put our kids through college, bought houses, bought cars, all because we've worked here so long, and he's been a big part of making it possible to work here so long." The president said, "I'm going to write him a thank-you note, and if any of you are interested in writing one, here's his contact information." About three weeks later, the hospital president happened to be at corporate headquarters and saw a pile of thank-you notes on the table in the CEO's office. The thank-you notes had such an impact on the CEO, he started writing a lot more thank-you notes himself.

Don't wait for someone to reward and recognize you before you reward and recognize them. Show appreciation for your boss, and not just on National Boss's Day. Drop a note to your boss thanking them for providing coaching, removing a barrier, and so on, because bosses like to be recognized as much as any other employee does. Rewarded and recognized behavior gets repeated.

All this is about making people feel cared for. It's about paying attention and noticing what you can do to make life better for others. Small gestures that say, "I notice how hard you work," and, "I know none of this is easy," mean the world to people. They create a multiplier effect. Gratitude and positivity will spread across the organization like the ripples a stone makes when you toss it into a pond.

I was talking to a person who reminded me that when she first started working for Studer Group, Karen Cook, RN, one of the long-term Studer key people, bought her a pair of slippers. She mentioned to her that you're in hotels a lot, you're on your feet a lot, and it's really important to take care of your feet. In fact, Karen bought every new person who came to work with her who traveled a pair of slippers.

The person who told me this story said not only did she appreciate those slippers, but this act of kindness had a huge impact on her. First of all, she felt really cared for, but also it taught her to notice the little things that she could do to make others feel appreciated. Often, we underestimate the impact our actions have. In reality, they can change someone's world for the better.

Here's the bonus: Making life better for others makes our *own* life better, too. Even as we ignite the flame for others, we rekindle our own flame if we have lost it, or stoke it even more if it's alive and well. Helping others connect to their calling also reconnects us to our own.

CHAPTER 16

Always Sweat the Small Stuff

In healthcare, we tend to get the big, difficult things right. That's great. But sometimes it's the small things that trip us up. Because healthcare is so complex, there are a million details that need to happen in the right order and in the right sequence for things to work. When we don't get the little things right, it keeps us from doing the big things effectively. This can lead to a lot of frustration. So, while of course we need be vigilant about the "big stuff"—the issues that directly connect to the quality of patient care and that save lives—we also need to sweat the small stuff.

As I have said throughout this book, the core characteristic of healthcare workers is their desire to be useful and helpful. In fact, that's why the balance of life is so hard for people in healthcare. When something gets in the way of their being as helpful and useful as they want to be, they can become frustrated. This may happen more often in healthcare than it does in most professions because of the sheer amount of details that must be handled and the tremendous drive people have to provide patients the best care.

When I talk about the "small stuff," I mean issues like scheduling and quick access to information, equipment not being available, communication not being as good as it could be, ineffective handoffs, and so forth. These are barriers that limit people and organizations from high performance. They keep us from being helpful and useful. Very often it's not the huge issues that trip people up but the small roadblocks. We are more likely to trip over a pebble than the Grand Canyon.

Knowing When to Tweak and When to Overhaul

We need to do all we can to prevent the circumstances that cause frustration. When systems and processes aren't working well for our physicians and staff, we need to rethink or sometimes overhaul them. Of course, the first step is knowing the difference between "we need to overhaul the entire system" and "this is a one-off or a temporary situation that doesn't require major changes, only minor tweaks."

When I was working with a large healthcare organization, they knew that periodically, for short time periods, they would be full, meaning no inpatient rooms would be available. Of course, you know how we are in healthcare. When we get full, we just buckle down and we handle it. It's hard but we deal with it. But we also know it's a short-term problem. So maybe we know this month or these two weeks will be tough. We understand when there's an accident, many, many people will be brought to the hospital all at once in a trauma-type situation, and we're going to deal with it. But if people know there is a light at the end of the tunnel, it improves morale.

The COVID-19 pandemic has shown us that no matter the circumstances, healthcare people buckle down and deal with it because that's how they are. They don't run away when the going gets tough. They're like firefighters: While everybody else is running away from the fire, they're running toward the fire.

Anyway, this hospital was in their normal period of being full. They'd done a lot of really good things to make them a better organization. The difference this time was the full capacity wasn't stopping. Two months turned into three months. Then three months turned into four months. The executive team was faced with a challenge because they didn't want to change systems or hire people if patient volume was going to go back down to normal levels.

It became apparent that they were running out of things like linens and other support mechanisms, because they were full for a longer time than usual. So then the question I posed to the administrative team was: When do you know it's not just a blip? When do you know it's going to be a consistent issue that needs to be managed?

This organization determined that if census stays at a certain level for a certain period of time, it would be considered a long-term issue rather than just a short-term issue. They looked at the numbers and said, "Okay. Our census is now going to run higher. We have a new normal, so we've got to beef up all the support mechanisms." That's an example of making sure the culture and the system supports the staff who are out there on the front lines, whether it's direct patient care or not, so those people can be helpful and useful.

Communicating Goes a Long Way.

If we determine that a system isn't running as well as it can, then we need to let people know we're going to fix it. When we can acknowledge the problem and narrate the situation, we can coach them through it. Sometimes just a little bit of communication goes a long way. We also need to let people know how long this will take. Often just knowing there's an end in sight makes a problem a lot more endurable.

Have you ever been in an organization and the elevator's broken, and there's a sign on it that reads, "Out of order"? I understand the elevator's not working, but what I really want to know is when will it be working?

Here is an example. A much-used elevator in a busy hospital wasn't working. If people didn't know it was broken, they would transport patients to it. Then they would realize it was broken and have to go to another bank of elevators. Eventually everyone stopped going to that elevator, not knowing when it would be fixed. So the staff created a technique to help. They basically said, "Let's include on the sign an estimate for when we think it will be fixed. Then people will know it's probably going to be broken at least till then so they'll quit going over there and trying it. They won't have to wonder."

Letting people know when the elevator will be fixed saves people time, and time is precious. It might not seem like a big deal to somebody not using the elevator, but if you're in patient care and that elevator is really important to you, you truly want to know when it is or isn't working (and if it's not working, when it's going to be fixed).

Those are examples of the techniques we think are small and unimportant, but they're really not. Again, no one trips over the Grand Canyon, but if you trip on those pebbles along the way, those can still cause injury. So, in healthcare, what we want to do is remove those pebbles as much as possible, so people can be as productive as possible.

How do we go about dismantling barriers? Part of it is understanding the value of clear, concise communication. Vagueness is a barrier. Clarity is vital to success. As mentioned earlier, the Heath brothers wrote in their book *Switch: How to Change Things When Change Is Hard* that 80 percent of failures are from a lack of clarity.[1] That's truly explaining exactly what the goal is, what right looks like, and what is taking place. When people know what to expect, they manage change so much better.

Engaging Others in Finding Solutions

Another important aspect of removing barriers is getting employees involved. Very often the person closest to the problem is the most likely to be able to solve it. People often don't realize they have the power to remove the barrier. When you coach people through situations and get them used to noticing problems and coming up with solutions—and rewarding and recognizing them for doing so—it can change a lot of things. What you're really doing is creating an empowered culture.

I've seen organizations that give Remove the Barrier Awards to people who recognize barriers and remove them. Sometimes we might not even realize there's a barrier in an organization. Because it's been there for so long, it just becomes normal, and people don't think it can be changed. The abnormal becomes normal. Once we get people used to looking for barriers and thinking about solving them, it's amazing how much improvement can happen.

One valuable tool is "coaching in the moment," which might also be called "on-the-spot" coaching. When we coach in the moment, we help people take ownership of removing the barriers that are tripping them up. A big part of this centers on helping people see how their job connects to the organizational big picture and to important outcomes. When they're able to see how their job ties back to how the organization functions, they can more easily find fixes that make sense.

In the past, I have written and spoken at length about a concept I describe as "Park Ranger Leadership." Basically, it's the attitude that leaders will swoop down and rescue people if they get "lost in the wilderness." Unfortunately, this discourages ownership and can prevent people from coming up with their own practical, workable solutions.

In healthcare, we get promoted because we are solution people, and that's wonderful. But if we always give someone a solution to their problem, we miss the opportunity to provide development. If somebody comes to me for a solution every single time they have a problem, they won't learn to find solutions on their own. If a person keeps getting lost in the woods and they keep running up to the park ranger asking for help, eventually the park ranger will say, "Why don't we work on helping you so you don't get lost?"

In healthcare, we have to be careful, because every time we give someone a solution—every time we walk that person out of the woods—we feel good about it, because we're being helpful and useful to that person. But we have to hold up the mirror and ask ourselves, *Am I being helpful long-term?* Being helpful short-term does not allow that person to learn on their own so they can evolve their own skill.

Here's an example of coaching in the moment and allowing staff to find their own solutions. A nursing unit was having trouble on their journey to accepting a higher daily census, so they talked to the nurse manager about it. This nurse manager in the past would have fixed the problem for them. Instead, she paused and said to her staff, "It seems like our census is going to be like this for a while. What are some changes we can make in order to address the census?" They'd already addressed the staffing issue, so she asked them for other suggestions for how they thought they could improve the situation. The staff quickly mentioned the need to adjust the current inventory levels for a number of items. The nurse manager said, "Great, let me know what you feel they should be."

This is on-the-spot coaching in that the manager helped the staff be part of the solution. On-the-spot coaching is not about embarrassing someone. Its purpose is to let staff know the leader trusts them to find their own solutions, receive input, and provide immediate feedback. It also helps people see challenges in a different way, prompting them to look a little deeper and diagnose more accurately what the real issue is.

Here is an example that shows how on-the-spot coaching gets people to evaluate and assess a situation differently. I was touring with the president of a hospital and heard one of the staff members say to the nurse executive that they were short-staffed.

The CEO asked the CNO, "Are we short-staffed, and if we are, how much are we?" We looked at the staffing and found out they weren't short-staffed at that time. So the question was, if on the metrics they're not short-staffed, why did they feel short-staffed? There are times when even if you hit the metrics, you're short-staffed at moments. They went back to the staff and said, "Gee. According to what we're seeing here, we do have the right staffing levels. Tell us why you're feeling short-staffed right now." That's what we really needed to figure out: "Why are you feeling that way right now?"

And they said, "Well, we've got these admits that just came up on the unit, and we're a little concerned because it seems like the shift before us stalled bringing them up, knowing that we would have to go through the admission process."

Now that was their perception. It probably happened only once in a while. They also said, "We've also been waiting for transport. Transport said they'd be up here 20 minutes ago, and they're still not here. So we've got these admissions coming in, and we have these transport issues."

So what that meant was, at that moment, they were absolutely right. They were short-staffed. But if the CEO and CNO had just accepted that without digging deeper into the issue, then it would have seemed like they were short-staffed for the whole shift. The on-the-spot coaching helped people to see that their assumption that they were short-staffed was really just a perception and not reality. So we had to develop process improvement techniques that we could put in place.

On-the-spot coaching is a great remedy for Park Ranger Leadership. It gets people in the habit of solving problems on their own rather than just bringing them to the leader. It forces them to think through what's frustrating them and to come up with their own recommendations. The immediacy of it makes it even more effective: A scenario that's unfolding in front of their eyes is a lot more meaningful than a theoretical one. And it truly shows people that they have the ability (and the permission) to make their own decisions in removing roadblocks.

Great employees really appreciate on-the-spot coaching. We're finding more and more that the number-one retention tool for an employee is development. Because in healthcare, people want to be effective. I've always been so impressed with physicians, nurses, and others who work in areas that require certification, because it means that a person has to get continuing education credits in their area of expertise in order to maintain their certification. On-the-spot coaching is a less formal, but no less powerful form of employee development.

Here's another example of on-the-spot coaching. I own a minor league baseball team. We have a young superstar who works for us named Daniel Venn, and he's in charge of media. We were getting ready to do a video he knew we were excited about, so he researched multiple videography firms and decided on the one he thought would be the best fit for our needs. He sent me an email asking if it was okay to sign the contract. I trusted Daniel's decision and agreed with signing the contract, but I also realize Daniel's young and although it would be great if he stayed with us forever, he's probably going to go work somewhere else at some point.

So I responded, "Daniel, I support the contract. However, for your own development, I think it's really important for you to send another email explaining to us why we should sign the contract. Why are you recommending this particular videography firm? You probably don't need to do this for this project, but I think it's important for your skill development and will really help you long-term in your career."

He sent his recommendations with a nice note, thanking me for the opportunity to develop. This was a confidence booster. This was his chance to make a big decision, and coaching reinforced that he had done it well.

With all the great benefits of this technique, we may miss the opportunity to coach in the moment? Maybe we're too rushed or feel that we have bigger things to deal with. But not only is this the perfect way to help people to learn in real time, it keeps bad habits from forming. Little issues that might be fixed with an on-the-spot conversation go unaddressed. Eventually, these little things grow into bigger things. This creates a multiplier effect. People don't improve, so the overall performance of the department doesn't progress. Results become harder to achieve. Your highest performing employees may end up leaving…and so forth.

Here are a few suggested techniques for on-the-spot coaching:

Walk them through the roadblock they're facing. This will help them see the real nature of the problem, rather than making assumptions that may or may not be accurate.

Rather than giving them a solution, ask, "What is your recommendation?" This teaches them to "own" solutions rather than always looking to leaders to provide them. People know more than they think they know. Asking them for their recommendation allows them to get the win.

Phrase things in a way that doesn't create defensiveness. For example, ask, "Is it okay if I give you feedback? I know you're very committed to your own professional development. Is it okay if I give you some feedback right now?" The majority of the time, the answer is yes. If not yes now, a time for feedback will be set.

You always want to give people an exit strategy so they don't feel trapped into a corner. Saying, "This is my perception, but I may be wrong; help me understand what's going on," can prevent defensiveness.

You also particularly want to let the person know that you're committed to their development, and you're doing this because you care about them as a person.

Finally, connect back to the larger *why*. As I mentioned, we need to remind the employee how their job ties into the bigger organizational picture. And that larger *why* is the patient experience.

When I started focusing on patient experience, there were no chief patient experience officers. There were very few people in organizational development. Today, many organizations have those individuals, which is absolutely great. Yet it does not mean others can back off. Everyone is in charge of organizational development, both in our own department and in the larger hospital or health system.

It's up to each one of us to look for and help remove the barriers that prevent the organization from providing the best possible patient experience. Sweating the small stuff is a crucial job. The well-being of our patients depends on it.

CHAPTER 17

Using Words That Connect to People's Values

Healthcare people are extremely values-driven. They tend to have solid values with few or no "gray" areas. That's a good thing. What it means for leaders is that when we are asking them to do something new, the words we use really matter. We need to say things in a way that connects to and resonates with their values. This is what motivates them to change their behavior.

I have learned this firsthand over the years. Often when I'm brought into a situation, it's because their results aren't exactly what they would want. In helping organizations change these results, I've learned how to use the words that matter most to my audience, much in the way the best clinicians use words the patient and family understand.

As my healthcare career progressed, I picked up words like *churn, revenue cycle, market basket, FTEs, EBITDA, vertical and horizontal integrating, capitation,* and so forth. There's nothing wrong with those words used at the right time. My problem was they became part of my daily language, and these words don't necessarily resonate with all audiences.

The goal is to use words that connect back to a person's values. Once we do this, even in the busiest times, they're going to do the right behavior to get the outcome. We no longer exist in a command-and-control environment, if we ever really did. We don't live in a do-it-because-I-told-you-to world. To achieve and sustain results requires connecting the dots for those who need to carry out the actions in a way that brings value to the work.

Over the years, I've visited many organizations to help improve their metrics across a variety of measurement systems. Each measurement system typically has its own lingo, and I find the words have crept into the vocabulary of the organization in a way that may or may not connect with the workforce.

When the results aren't good, there are many reasons given. No one wants to say, "We're not trying." They *are* trying. No one's going to say, "We don't care," because people do care.

So why aren't people doing certain behaviors? The following story illustrates why certain behaviors aren't done, and what can happen when we don't link to people's values.

I was meeting with a group of emergency department staff a healthcare system had brought together, as well as some charge nurses, managers, chief nursing officers, vice presidents of nursing, patient care, and so forth. They were frustrated with their patient experience results.

I said, "Help me understand the ER a little better. Let's talk about some reasons a patient comes to the ER. Let's say I have chest pains and I come to the ER. Tell me what happens." Of course, they immediately walked through the protocol they would follow if I were a patient having chest pains. I asked what they would do if a patient had been in an accident and was in shock. Again, they walked me through what they would do. I used the example of the time my wife fell and shattered her kneecap, and it was the same story. These clinicians knew their stuff.

It was very obvious how committed they were to making sure patients got what they considered the best clinical care. Then I said, "What if, when I came to the ER with chest pains, you had an interim nurse manager? Would you still follow the same protocols?" They said, "Absolutely." Then I asked, "What if you were staffed a little light that day? Would you still follow the protocol?" Again, they answered, "Absolutely." "What if you were really busy?" Same answer.

I gave a number of examples. Every time they looked at me and said, "We'd still do these things." I asked, "Why would you still do these things?" And they said, "Well, because if we didn't, the patient wouldn't have the best clinical outcome."

Then it hit me: The reason they weren't doing some other things to improve patient experience was because we, leadership, did not connect those acts to clinical outcomes. Once people believe their actions will help the patient, even in the most difficult situations, the proper action will be taken.

On the inpatient side, I am not confident all staff get excited about raising HCAHPS scores. HCAHPS scores may not motivate everyone. But what all clinicians *can* unite behind is helping the patient understand the side effects of medication, helping them understand their discharge plans, and so on.

We can connect HCAHPS to the quality of care, and hospitals that raise their HCAHPS results tend to have better clinical outcomes.

When people understand this, they will engage on a deeper level. They will understand that when patient experience results move, so do safety measures and clinical outcomes. It becomes a matter of values. And once we've connected to their values, they will make sure to implement the tactics that improve the results. And if an employee sees someone *not* doing a tactic, they'll be more likely to speak up.

It's the same thing with almost everything we do in an organization. If we can weave it back to how this impacts something that's important to their values, people can't *not* do it. A lot of people value their commitment to coworkers (i.e., "If I don't do this, my coworker's going to pay the price, and I'm a good team player."). For physicians, the bottom line is always going to be creating the best clinical outcomes for patients.

In 2015, I coauthored a book with Dr. George Ford entitled *Healing Physician Burnout.* Over 90 percent of the book focuses on how to create the right culture for doctors. A single chapter deals with well-being suggestions physicians can control. A portion of this chapter was devoted to self-care, with an even smaller portion about issues like stress management. There are a few paragraphs on meditation. Why did we include so little about self-care relative to culture-building? Because the goal was to speak the physicians' language.

I am a big believer in mindfulness. I do transcendental meditation. It is very effective. The main point is it helps to resolve the triggers that create anxiety. However, for physicians, it's sort of like telling somebody at an airport every time the plane's delayed because of mechanical problems, "Will you just go over there and meditate for a while?" What they probably want to say is, "Well, I'll go meditate, but it would really be good if you could just get the planes running on time." Creating that right culture is what physicians really care about. And why? Because if we create the right culture for physicians, it is more efficient. If they're more efficient and effective, they can impact clinical outcomes. It leads to physicians' feeling respected.

When we learn what drives a person, we can deliberately choose words that connect to their values. When we can connect back to values, then the people are compliant not because they're told to be compliant; they do the behavior because it connects back to why this makes sense. As a manager or a leader, we've got to clarify what the end result is. If we can help people understand the end result, it really pays dividends.

As I shared earlier, at Baptist Hospital people would come to benchmark us. We would provide them a schedule, and at the end of the day, we'd get together and we'd ask them what they thought. We would also ask them to share one of their own best practices that we could learn from so it would be a mutually beneficial day.

A vice-president of one of the hospitals that came to visit us admitted that he broke away from the schedule because he wanted to find out on his own. So he went out into the parking lot, ran into a security guard, and asked, "What do you think of this focus the administration has on patient satisfaction?" (That's what we talked about, the patient experience or patient perception of care, at the time.) The security guard said, "Well, from what I understand, if we make our patients and their families feel a lot better, more people will come here. The more people who come here, the better the organization does. The better the organization does, the more secure my job is, and job security is very important to me and my family. It makes sense to me." That clicked it for the VP; that security guard in the parking lot had connected the dots.

Here is another example of connecting to people's values. A hospital dressed their housekeeping staff in clinical clothes versus what would normally be environmental clothes. They saw housekeepers as clinicians, and told them, "When you help keep this place clean, we have fewer infections." Not only did they connect their words to the hospital staff's values, they connected their actions to those values. The clothing they provided spoke volumes.

Before we end this chapter, I'd like to share a time I learned a lesson about using the right words the hard way.

When people come to the emergency room for some reason—for example, a broken ankle—they might have other health issues unrelated to their ankle. It makes sense to do a quick assessment to find out if the patient has gone to the doctor recently. Have they had certain diagnostic tests that they should be having at their age? So we started adding quick health assessment questions when appropriate with patients in the emergency room.

One of the assessments was regarding mammograms. It was amazing how many people came to the emergency room for other issues who could have had a mammogram and had not. We started asking, "Would you like us to schedule a mammogram?" There was no pressure other than wanting to improve a person's health. It was working great. Our women's center suddenly started exceeding revenue projections. We were doing more mammograms than we had ever done.

I got so excited about it, I decided to stop into the women's center to congratulate them. I said, "Congratulations, we have broken our volume record. We've done more mammograms this month than ever before." And they looked at me. They were nice and polite but not near as excited about it as I was. Now you might be thinking, *You've got to be kidding me. You used those words?* The answer is yes.

I could tell my comments landed flat. I thought about it over the next few days and realized volume is not what excites them; it's not why they're in healthcare. They're in healthcare to help people detect whether they have cancer or not, which means a patient can leave relieved or hopefully they can catch it as soon as possible. We did research on how many mammograms were positive and how many were success stories. Dr. Rubey shared that if they catch the cancer early, the treatment is much less difficult for the patient.

I went back to the women's center and said, "I want to apologize for coming in and talking about volume. I used the wrong word. I want to thank you. This last month, you helped more people than ever before either identify they didn't have cancer or catch it earlier than they would have, because you did such a professional job in the breast cancer care center here. Thank you." I then shared what Dr. Rubey had told me. And this time the response was completely different.

When we can connect our words to a behavior that the employee or the physician knows is going to have a positive impact on a patient, a coworker, or themselves, we connect to their values. And once we plug into a person's values, they want to take the actions we're asking them to take—and the actions are consistent. They see what we are asking them to do as a necessary part of living up to their calling.

Using the words that connect to people's values is how we achieve compliance. And once we get compliance, we get consistency. When we get consistency across an organization, we can achieve and sustain great performance. Consistency and sustainability are two characteristics of values-driven organizations. It's amazing to consider how much we can achieve when we begin by using the right words!

CHAPTER 18

How Great Communication Creates Consistency, Engagement, and Alignment

The most effective leaders are usually the best communicators. They have to be. We work in such complex, fast-moving environments that it takes great skill to cut through the chaos and share information in a way that not only gets "heard" but motivates people to act. No wonder when reviewing employee engagement surveys, we consistently find *communication* is one of the top items that could be improved. This is true even when we think communication is quite good.

Being able to provide consistent, well-thought-out, real-time communication is one of the most crucial leadership competencies. Along with training, good communication is what pushes responsibility and authority to the front lines. This is so important in a hospital, where we have to act quickly and decisively.

Great communication fills emotional bank accounts. When we handle communication the right way—even when we're asking people to make incredibly tough changes—we can actually strengthen relationships and positively impact the entire organization.

The right kind of communication alleviates anxiety and keeps people from feeling overwhelmed. It keeps people engaged and connected (to each other and to their sense of purpose). It keeps organizations aligned and on the same page, nimble, adaptive, and able to innovate. Great communication is the oil that keeps the machine running smoothly.

For all of these reasons, organizations need to get intentional about communication and make it a priority. Get crystal clear on the information you want shared, and hardwire mechanisms that allow you to cascade messages throughout the organization. This is the only way to make sure the right messages reach everyone.

Communication is a huge topic. It would be easy to write a book (a long book!) on all the facets. For now, let's just look at a few tips I have seen be successful.

Ask What Right Looks Like to Them.

Here's how this works. Each leader meets with their direct reports. Start the meeting by saying: "Let's decide what excellent communication looks like. We know we want excellent communication, so tell me what it looks like to you." Then go around the room and hear from each person. This exercise will be interesting, because some who have rated communication as not being that great will likely struggle to define excellent communication.

The great thing about this method is that it gets everyone on the same page regarding communication. You might need to keep urging them to clarify what they feel is lacking. For instance, they might say, "Well, we just want to know what's going on." You could then respond by saying, "Well, let's talk about a time that we had really good communication." And then, "Tell me something that wasn't communicated well or in a timely way, so we can stop those types of situations." And then move into, "Tell me what information you would like."

Then, after everyone has had a chance to share their thoughts, you will say: "Now here's some information we, as an organization, want you to have. These are goals of progress that we want everyone to understand and be aware of." Clarify what those are and explain why they are important. Then ask the group, "How do you think you should get this communication? Should you get it via email? Should we post it somewhere?" The group then gets to decide, as a department, how it's going to be provided.

Here's the beauty of this: After all the topics above have been discussed and everyone has articulated their preferences, it's time to say, "Now that we have agreed on how you want to receive these vital communications, can we also agree that it's your responsibility to read the messages and act on them?" Since they have had so much input into creating the process, there should be no reason for them to say no.

Finally, ask them, "How are we going to make sure people access the communication?" And then ask them, "What should we do with those employees who refuse to keep up-to-date on the communication?" These questions, along with the answers they provoke, really create accountability.

So, what are our wins when we take this approach? One, the entire team gets clarification on what excellent communication looks like. Two, leaders get a commitment from the staff to be accountable for reading the communication. This, in particular, is a huge win in an organization. And for managers, it provides a sense of relief because now they are not trying to hit a vague target.

Fixing the Sequencing Challenge

A big communication issue is that people across the organization hear vital information at different times. A senior leader meets with direct reports to share information that needs to be cascaded. Then those leaders meet with *their* direct reports on wildly varying time tables. As a result, certain people end up learning the vital information later than others. They think, *Why am I the last to know?* Or they end up hearing it secondhand from someone else. The key is to cascade information in a way that everyone hears the information at the same time.

I remember sitting with a group of leaders and asking the top leader, "When do you meet with your direct reports?" And he told me, "Every Tuesday from 9:00 to 11:00 a.m." I said, "Great." Next, I went around the room and said to each leader, "So when you have this information, tell me when you then take it to the people who work for you."

Each person in the group then shared when they meet with their direct reports. One said, "Well, I meet every Thursday afternoon." Another one said, "I have a smaller area, so I usually do it individually." Another person said, "I meet once a month. It's the third Friday of every month." Another person said, "After this meeting, I meet Tuesday afternoon with my people." This went on until everyone had responded. When the CEO saw the sequence, I could tell he realized right away that even great communication can be seen as not great due to timing.

At the meeting, the decision was made that everyone would have a meeting at the same time to cascade the information from that meeting. The good news is that if, let's say, you needed to meet with everyone virtually or in person, that time is already slotted. So at the meeting, you could say, "This is so important. We think instead of having eight different cascades, we could do it all at one time."

Standardize the Talking Points You Want Shared.

A big challenge with communicating to groups is that not everyone hears what we say the same way. Often, we say so much that people may not recognize which points are the most important. This is why when we share information that's meant to be cascaded, we standardize the talking points. Consistency is everything. To make sure we get it, we need to be sure we clarify it and disseminate it across the organization the right way.

When I was president of a hospital, I wanted to check out how I was doing with my communication. So after a meeting, I asked people to send me the top three talking points that they took out of the meeting. There were probably 80 or 90 people in that room and we covered many different key points. I discovered that many times, people identified the most important one but then their answers would vary on key points two and three. Now, they also can always add points specific to their department or unit, but in this exercise I was looking for the bullet points we wanted everyone to recognize. It was my fault for not clarifying the bullet points to cascade to others.

We need to make sure the key message points are not missed. It helps to pause after each agenda item has been discussed. In between agenda items, you can even say, "Pause." Attendees will ask questions, at which point you can decide whether those questions need to be rolled out outside of this meeting. If the answer is no, just go right to the next agenda item. If it is yes, then you can ask, "Okay, so what are the bullet points we're going to roll out? Who's going to roll them out? When and how are they going to roll out?"

These are just a few simple tools that can move your communication from being sporadic and scattershot to being unified and consistent. Imagine how much more effective your organization will be when everyone is hearing the same messages at the same time. And imagine how much more engaged and less anxious people will be when there is clarity around what they are supposed to do.

Communication is how work gets done. *Great* communication is a force multiplier. It makes everything you do more impactful...and over time, it accelerates your performance.

CHAPTER 19

Words Matter: How the Right Words Relieve Anxiety and Shape the Patient Experience

Words matter in every industry, but in healthcare, they can make a profound difference in people's lives. In fact, they may determine how people experience the most critical moments they will ever face. The words we choose can heal or harm patients, motivate or confuse them, soothe them or stress them out.

Not only do we need to make sure patients clearly understand what we are telling them, we need to carefully consider the emotional impact of our words. We need to make sure our words convey empathy, that they say to the patient, "I see where you are right now and I want to make this difficult experience as easy as possible." We need to be so careful about the role we play in shaping a moment that will be remembered forever.

Sometimes in healthcare we may have to give people terrible news about a loved one. When I talk to doctors about what it's like to deliver such a tough message, they say that while it is so, so hard, it's also a privilege to help people navigate some of the worst moments of their lives. This is why I believe healthcare is truly a calling. Not everyone can do this work. It takes a special kind of person.

I love Dr. Stephen Beeson. Over the years, we have collaborated in many areas. He shared a story with me about having to tell a woman that she had terminal cancer. As he told the story, he kept reflecting on the fact that the husband and he were about the same age. The couple's children were about the same age as his children. And the woman he was telling she would not be there to raise her children was about the same age as his wife. I can only imagine the empathy with which he delivered the news.

I've heard him tell this story numerous times, and he starts to get teary-eyed each time he recalls the experience. I have found that's a common thread with many of us, that there are certain events we've gone through in healthcare, that no matter how many times we tell the story, we relive the experience over and over again. Discomfort is something we live with in healthcare, but that doesn't make it pleasant, and we certainly wish we could avoid it.

I read a book by Dr. Anthony Orsini about having difficult conversations. It is titled *It's All in the Delivery: Improving Healthcare Starting With a Single Conversation.* Dr. Orsini certainly knows a lot about difficult conversations because he has had to have many of them. He's a physician in a neonatal intensive care unit, so he's had to tell families the baby they looked so forward to taking home would never come home. The loss of a child is something no family would ever want to go through. His book does a really nice job of framing those conversations and teaching how to deliver some of the toughest messages of all.

The reason I like the Orsini book is because training is so crucial in this area. In healthcare we often get more focused on the clinical side of what we do every day, but the emotional side is just as important. Sometimes we learn from formal training, but usually we learn from watching a coworker or supervisor do it, or we just figure it out ourselves. *It's All in the Delivery* is a great guide for those of us who need to teach ourselves or others how to have these tough conversations.

I have so much respect for folks who deliver hard news well. They have a gift for making things better for the patient. Everything about them conveys how much they care. That's what patients really want to know.

When we work in a hospital, there are so many opportunities for us to make a difference in people's lives. The key is remembering the patient's state of mind. When we work in a medical environment day in and day out, it's easy to underestimate the anxiety patients feel. We need to remember that for most people hospitals are scary places. Anything we can do that shows the patient that we're highly competent and that we care will go a long way toward relieving their anxiety.

The Power of Words

Key words at key times make a difference. Some of those were put into the acronym AIDET.® It is a simple tool that helps providers showcase their competency, experience, and caring in a way that reduces patient anxiety, makes them feel better, and allows them to take an active role in their care. All of this improves outcomes. Many organizations accomplish the same results with their own acronyms. The acronyms work if staff are part of developing them.

AIDET walks the healthcare provider through the following steps:

Acknowledge. We acknowledge the patient by name if at all possible, and we acknowledge the family members if they're there.

Introduce. We introduce ourselves, our skill set, and our experience. When we let people know, for example, that we've done a procedure hundreds of times, it naturally reduces their anxiety.

Duration. This means describing a test and letting the patient know how long it will take before the results come back. It means letting them know how long it will be before they get a bed, or receive pain medication, or get to go home.

Explanation. The more you explain what's going to happen and why, the less anxious the patient will be. Uncertainty creates anxiety. Explanation relieves it. Also, the more you explain, the more compliant the patient will be—and the more compliant they are, the better their outcomes will be.

Thank you. "Thank you for choosing our hospital."[1]

Over the years, I have found that certain key words reduce anxiety, not just in patients but also in employees and any human being.

Sometimes when we are providing information to employees on how to use AIDET, they struggle a little. Remembering all five letters can feel overwhelming to people who are really busy. Yes, it's meant to be a system and it all works well together, but it might be too much for some people to learn all at once. It may help to have staff implement one letter at a time until they master it and get their confidence up. Then, move on to the next letter.

In the past, I've found the letter that caused the most pushback was the letter "I." Many people have said, "I'm just not comfortable because I feel like I'm bragging about myself."

I can see that. Nobody wants to sit here and say, "Let me tell you how great I am." In the normal world, that is true, but the healthcare world is a high-anxiety environment. People are hearing every bleep and seeing every wire on the machine they're hooked up to. They are also trying to understand so much they may miss things their provider said. The goal of the "I" is to help patients and their families feel less anxious.

The challenge with getting people to use the "I" is to get them through the discomfort of feeling like they are bragging. We find the best way to do it is to role model the situation. For instance, in training, I would say, "If you're coming in for a mammogram and the technologist says, 'I'm going to be helping with your mammogram,' how much confidence would you have in that person? How about if the technologist says, 'I'm a licensed radiologic technologist and I have additional training in mammograms. I've done over 8,000 mammograms, and I'm going to do everything I can to make this as comfortable as possible. With any mammogram, there could be discomfort, but with my experience, I will make it the very best it can be.'" Then I would ask, "Which of these would you prefer to do your mammogram?" They always picked the latter.

It really helps when leaders model AIDET. We have also found it helps when the manager role models exactly what they're asking the staff to do. That way the staff sees the impact in real time. Also, role playing can help. We'd set up labs and have people practice AIDET. The more we practice, the more confidence we build, and the easier it gets. Also, reversing the roles, where employees get to be the patient, really shows them how it feels to hear the words.

Practicing AIDET might be uncomfortable at first. This is when we need to emphasize that there are many actions and behaviors that may seem uncomfortable but that do improve outcomes. When people realize this, their values won't let them not do it.

What I Learned About Effective Communication on the Other Side of AIDET

I have my own personal experience with how much of a difference the right words make when a loved one is a patient. My own son Michael was in an accident in July of 1995 at a campground in Deadwood, South Dakota.

On a Friday afternoon, the day before we were set to leave, my wife and one of my daughters decided to take a swim in the pool, and my son and I were kicking a soccer ball. Around 3:00 p.m., I was going to call Holy Cross Hospital, and since I did not have a cell phone then, I went to the payphone at the campground. I asked my wife to watch Mike and I put him inside the fence at the swimming pool. While I was on the phone, the ball got kicked over the fence. I'm sure my wife told him not to go outside the fence, but he either couldn't hear her or was anxious to get the ball. A gentleman was on a 4,800-pound Bobcat moving some dirt off a road where the ball went. My son went to pick it up. The Bobcat went in reverse and crushed him.

I was in the campground building and a gentleman ran in and said, "Call 911! A little boy's been crushed." And, I don't know why, but I knew that was my son. I rushed out and there was pandemonium. My wife was leaning over our son saying, "There's no heartbeat. There's no pulse." My son was gray. It was just a blur. It seemed like in a matter of minutes, the ambulance pulled up. The paramedics said Mike had a heartbeat and they put him in the ambulance. My wife hopped in the ambulance with them. I jumped in our minivan with my daughter, and we went to the first hospital, a critical access hospital, which is why I loved them so much. They stabilized him, and then they said, "We're going to transfer him to a larger hospital in Rapid City." My wife hopped in the ambulance again, and my daughter and I hopped in the van. They beat us to the hospital.

When I got to the hospital, Mike was already in the pediatric intensive care unit. When I walked in his room, my son had all these wires in him—it was a mess. He was bleeding internally, his rib cage was into his heart, his shoulder had damage, and he was on morphine. My wife was in there with him. I put my daughter in the waiting room, went into my son's room, and said to my wife, "Is Michael going to live?" And she said yes. Now, I don't think she had any clinical reason to say that, except in her mother's heart she needed to believe it, as we all did. I started asking her questions, and she said, "The doctor's down the hallway." I went to see the doctor and introduced myself. For some reason I told him I worked in healthcare. I asked him if my son would live, and he said, "We don't know right now. The next 24 to 36 hours will be critical."

I was so scared. If your child might not live, which hospital do you want him in? I asked the doctor in the nicest way possible, "Where'd you go to medical school?" He must have known exactly why I asked, because he said, "I went to the University of Michigan. I did a residency in pediatric medicine. Then I did a fellowship in intensive care. I am double board certified in intensive care and pediatrics. The reason I'm here is because I grew up here and I wanted to come back to my hometown." I went into my son's room, looked at my wife, and said, "We got lucky. He's in a great place." Was that doctor giving me, a father of a child who was in critical condition, confidence that my son was in the right place? Absolutely. Did it reduce my anxiety? It didn't reduce my anxiety about my son's condition, but it did reduce my anxiety about who was taking care of him.

About nine days later, we were discharged from the hospital. Today my son is in his thirties and he's fine. So, a small hospital in Deadwood, South Dakota, and a large hospital in Rapid City showed me the power of the "I," but I didn't realize it then.

Through the years in my work, there have been many things people found to be a little bit uncomfortable, and AIDET has been one of them. But I hear so many great stories on its impact that it makes the initial discomfort worth it.

On one occasion, a number of physicians at an organization had been presented a session on the use of AIDET. I was there to speak several weeks after the sessions with physicians had been concluded. Before I spoke, they wanted me to talk to one of the doctors. The doctor said that when he left the training in AIDET some months back, he thought it was phony—a guest relations tidbit. He told me he tried it just to show it wouldn't work.

The first patient who came in was a patient he was seeing for the first time. He told the patient where he went to medical school, residency, fellowship, and that he'd been treating thousands of cancer patients for 22 years. He said before he got finished, the patient and their family started crying because they felt they were in the right place. He thought that maybe that was just a fluke. But the fourth patient started crying as well. He said by the end of that first day practicing the "I," he wanted to cry because he had missed an opportunity for these 22 years to help his patients feel less anxious and more secure that they were in the right place.

That's how powerful the right words can be. And it's why we have a human responsibility to use them every chance we get.

CHAPTER 20

Understanding and Appreciating Differences

Healthcare has amazing facilities and the latest in state-of-the-art equipment that they are really proud of, but if you ask any leader, they will tell you their most valuable asset is their people. People are what make hospitals great, and how they work together as a team to help provide patient care is really important.

There is probably no other place besides healthcare where you will find more people with diverse backgrounds, education, specialties, temperaments, and personalities working together. (It really is a bit of a hodge-podge!) And all of these people are doing incredibly important work on a seemingly impossible schedule.

It's these individual differences that make us so strong as an organization. Still, sometimes these personality differences can create problems for us. Each of us perceives and processes information differently, and those differences show up in our work habits.

In healthcare, we've always been committed to learning and getting better and better. It's an ongoing process. So it's no surprise that one area of this learning centers on how all the different personalities can work together most effectively. To figure out how to bring individual strengths and talents together to complement each other—so that the whole is greater than the sum of the parts—organizations often invest in assessments. These simple tools can be very telling.

At Baptist Hospital we decided to take the Myers-Briggs Type Indicator. This is a self-report questionnaire designed to identify an individual's personality type, strengths, and psychological preferences in how they make decisions. It was interesting, because when we announced that every person in leadership was going to take the Myers-Briggs, one of our physicians was very nervous about it. I'm sure there were others who were nervous too, but he was willing to speak up about it.

He was concerned about who would see the results. We made sure we told everyone that others wouldn't be able to see their results. There are no right or wrong answers in the Myers-Briggs personality inventory. You can't fail. But I think most of us are afraid of the unknown. Maybe some were worried that certain personality types were less desirable in some way and they would be labeled negatively. Of course this is not true, but as Jack Canfield said, F.E.A.R. stands for **F**anta-sized **E**xperiences **A**ppearing **R**eal.

We had a wonderful person come in and administer the Myers-Briggs. I didn't understand the results at that time. For those of you who may be wondering, I'm an ESTJ. This stands for Extraverted, Sensing, Thinking, Judging. My personality type tends to be goal-oriented and decisive. We don't mind making tough decisions and taking action. In fact, sometimes we tend to jump into action a bit too quickly.

The test administrator then sat us all at tables in groups of about eight. We didn't know it at the time, but she had grouped the same or similar personality types together. Then we got an assignment.

The facilitator said, "You've just been given as much money as you can possibly spend, and you have one week. What would you do?" My group, goodness, we were already in a plane, then we'd figure out where we were going. We assumed all the tables would come up with the same scenario we did. But when we started reporting our answers, some groups were wondering who was going to watch their cat, their dog, their house. Heck, my group forgot we even had a cat or a dog. We were up in the plane heading out.

It was so amazing. It really showcased our differences. What we learned was how to appreciate and respect the differences in people and how those differences can make us stronger as an organization.

Then we dug a little deeper. We started looking to see if there were jobs that tended to attract a certain personality type. Of course what we found doesn't apply to everyone, but we noticed there were certain professions that attracted more introverts and others where there were more extraverts. Many scientific people who major in chemistry and biology are drawn to healthcare—physicians in particular—and they tend to be more internally oriented. Again, this is not to say that all physicians are introverts. We just found that doctors were more likely to be introverted than extraverted. We'll talk more about why this matters later.

It went so well the physician who had initially been so concerned suggested we put the Myers-Briggs letters on our name badges so we could learn to better understand each other.

So How Does This Stuff Manifest?

The Myers-Briggs Personality Types are made up of four dimensions:

Extraversion (E) or Introversion (I). This dimension has to do with where you put your energy and attention: the outer world or the inner world. Are you energized and excited by being around people and doing lots of activities, or do you like a lot of alone time to reflect and recharge?

Sensing (S) or Intuition (N). How do you process information? Through your five senses (more step by step and fact-based) or through the impressions you receive (more concerned with big pictures, themes, and meaning)?

Thinking (T) or Feeling (F). How do you make decisions? Do you first take a more logical approach based on pros and cons and consequences, or do you focus more on values, how other people might be affected, and what's best for all?

Judging (J) or Perceiving (P). This dimension has to do with how you organize your life. Are you more of a planner, scheduler, and list-maker? Or do you prefer to be more flexible, adaptable, and spontaneous?

Of course this is a brief and broad explanation. A lot has been written on Myers-Briggs types, and if you're interested, I highly recommend doing some reading. It's fascinating stuff. You might want to start at www.myersbriggs.org.

Here is an example of how my personality type manifests. As an extravert, I am an external thinker. I can often recognize when somebody else is an external thinker. We just start talking. While we're talking, we might even compliment ourselves (e.g., I might say, "Well, that was good. Anybody write down what I just said?") because we think out loud. Our idea of a good time is to throw out a whiteboard and start brainstorming.

The challenge with that is we scare the heck out of the people who aren't like us, because they might be thinking, *Do they have any idea what they're saying or what they sound like?* We can also misjudge people. For example, because I will jump into a conversation, I might assume somebody who doesn't jump right in is not that engaged, which could be completely wrong. They might just want more time to think about it and understand it.

Because there's a big difference in the way people with different personalities think, there are different styles of work. For example, if you're a physician and you're a strong "I," you're probably focused on one patient at a time. If somebody who is a strong "E" comes up on the unit and they have three or four more patients they need to talk about, they just start talking. The introvert is thinking, *Can't you see I'm focusing on this one patient?* and the extravert is thinking, *Don't they realize they're ignoring me?* Both people may think the other is being rude but that is not the intention. They just have different styles of working and interacting with others.

We are different people with different personalities, and we have to learn to appreciate each other. Years ago our administrative group was getting ready to meet with a group of physicians. We had come up with some ways to reduce costs and had budgeted how much of a cost savings there would be once we reduced some standing orders. We were pretty pumped as we went into this medical staff meeting. As we rolled out the change in standing orders, right away the physicians started questioning it. In the end, we did not get approval to change the standing orders.

Of course, we went into our offices in administration and talked about how terrible it was that the doctors were blocking this. The physicians probably went off to one of their breakrooms and said, "Can you imagine administration trying to jam this down our throats?" And they were right. We learned a lesson from the Myers-Briggs assessment and found out we couldn't make a change that way. Out of respect for others, we needed to give the doctors time to think about things. There's one organization we worked with that whenever they were considering a change, unless it was an emergency, they gave everyone 30 days to study it, look at it, and ask questions. We found that when they met on it, it went way better than what we were doing.

Because of this, one of the things I recommend to any organization is to make sure a meeting agenda is out 24 hours ahead of time if possible. I'm not talking about emergent situations, but normal situations. If the agenda is out 24 hours ahead of time, that's respectful, because some people prefer to study the agenda so they can be better prepared for the meeting. By giving more time to those individuals who don't think out loud, we can achieve 100 percent involvement in a meeting instead of maybe only 50 percent.

While we used Myers-Briggs, there are lots of quality assessments out there that are rather inexpensive, easy to administer, and the results are easy to understand. They are simple but powerful tools that you can start to utilize immediately.

Another one we use at Studer Community Institute is Management By Strengths (MBS). It helps us determine people's temperaments by zeroing-in on four traits: Directness, Extraversion, Pace, and Structure. When we can understand people's temperaments, we can figure out how to leverage their strengths, improve communication with them, work more productively with them, build stronger teams, and so on.

MBS shows that there are four basic preferences: results- or outcome-oriented, team- or people-oriented, timing- or process-oriented, and detail- or structure-oriented. We all have a bit of each preference. The MBS provides to what degree we have each preference.

People love this. They put their colored graphs on their office doors, name tags, etc. One construction company even put it on their hard hats. One really helpful thing about knowing your preferences as well as your coworkers' is you can receive tips on how to best work with other people based on those preferences. Self-awareness and recognizing others' work styles creates magic in the organization and the respect that we're all looking for. By knowing people's strengths, we can place them in areas of the organization where they can flourish and balance out others around them.

I am not naturally a structured person, but I have learned that I need structure to succeed, so I surround myself with people who bring a lot of structure to my team. I like to hardwire systems and processes, because hardwiring makes things always happen the same way and keeps them consistent, which then achieves the desired outcome. I also need outcome-oriented people on my team because they are good at bringing clarity to goal-setting and can help drive the timelines. An organization works best when people with different personalities and work styles contribute to a common goal.

How Assessments Can Make Your Organization Stronger

Assessment tools can be incredibly valuable. Here are just some of the ways these assessments can help you be a better-run organization. They can:

Lessen frustration and conflict. We perceive and process information differently, and those differences show up in our work habits. Once we know and understand how someone might perceive or process information, we learn to adjust our communication to help get things done.

Spark personal growth in your staff and leaders. Understanding how you operate in the world and how others experience you can be an eye-opener. This kind of training can lead to more self-awareness and self-reflection. Self-awareness is needed for us to be coachable, and self-awareness and coachability are two of the most valuable qualities in leaders. Not only do assessments help us learn more about ourselves, they help us learn to recognize, understand, and appreciate how others are different.

Help you build better teams. When you know how each member of your team likes to work and whom they are most likely to collaborate with, you become more effective as an organization. You can build teams from people whose various strengths complement each other and counteract each others' weaknesses.

Improve communication. Once you know someone's personality type or preferences, you know how they process information and how they work best. You know how best to approach them and you will better understand how they respond to things.

Help you manage and motivate people. Some people work best with minimal feedback. Others may want lots of interaction. Not everyone is motivated by the same things.

Diversity is a wonderful thing. If everyone worked the same way; thought the same way; and had the same strengths, weaknesses, temperaments, and preferences, organizations would be greatly unbalanced. Imagine if everyone talked and brainstormed nonstop and there was nobody who would sit down and execute a plan? Or if you had a whole organization full of "executers" and no creative types to infuse fresh ideas? When everyone can see the value of differences, they will appreciate their coworkers more. That can only be a good thing.

Finally, understanding differences in people helps us do a better job of coaching, mentoring, and developing them. It's the gateway to real engagement, which is a key to retention, productivity, trusting relationships, positivity, and all the other things that make an organization great.

CHAPTER 21

How Frontline People and Middle Managers Drive Culture

I was speaking at an organization one time, and they announced that they were going to implement the tools and techniques I was going to present. As it turns out, this announcement was not well received. In fact, a cartoon was shared around the hospital that featured a graveyard of tombstones. All of the tombstones were inscribed with various initiatives that had failed over the years. And there with a fresh plot of dirt was a tombstone with my name on it.

It wasn't the most thrilling reception I've ever gotten at an organization. So, I asked to meet with the ringleaders. They spent a day and a half going through the workshop, and afterward they came up and apologized. What they mentioned was that there had just been so many failed programs. Naturally they assumed that this one would also fail.

This used to happen quite a bit inside organizations. People would get their hopes up with a new initiative, and then the new actions would not last. You would see that glassy-eyed look of, "Oh my gosh, here we go again. They're spending a lot of money on a consultant that would have been better being used here in our own organization. Give me the shirt, give me a slice of pizza, tell me the jargon, and call me in three years!"

The good news is that as I shared our framework and tactics, I began to find more and more people and organizations were getting quite good at executing them. I would ask employees, "How do you know something is different this time?"

This is the first answer I consistently heard: "We see our leader a lot more in our work area. Instead of being gone all the time at meetings, they are on the unit more."

Second, they'd say, "There are some things that we've been asking for or about for a long time. Well, it finally happened." (This could be a piece of equipment, or a better way of communicating, or a better process.)

The third thing I'd hear was, "Some of the people who were really difficult are no longer working here."

But the most significant change people noticed was that employees started to own a big part of the process. We know the culture is going to hold when peers coach peers. The magic you're looking for happens when an experienced person says to a newer person, "This is how we do it here." Or, "No, we don't do it that way here."

Often, I have felt that whoever has the strongest middle management team will have the best organization overall and the best chance to sustain the gains when changes are made. It's important for middle managers to own the culture. That's because executive leaders are more likely to move on than middle managers and frontline workers are.

With many large systems, senior leaders are asked to move to other locations. Early on, I shared with my wife, "For me to go to the next step in my career, it will likely mean relocating." It happened. We did relocate, then we relocated one more time.

On the other hand, middle management and frontline workers usually stay at an organization for a long time. They grew up in the community, their family lives there, their relatives live there, their high school friends live there. They're just less likely to relocate. As a result, they are pivotal to making sure everyone has what they need to live up to their calling and do their job. So the challenges of any senior management team is to hardwire a great system for high performance and create the strongest possible middle management team to execute on that system. And the goal of managers is to develop those frontline workers.

No senior executive wants to work so hard to build an organization that's high performing and leave and then find out a year or two later that things have eroded. They, too, are called. They are passionate about creating a great organization and they don't want its fate to depend on their presence. Quite the opposite. In the words of Lao Tzu, "An expert craftsman leaves no mark."

I went to speak at an organization, and the CEO had done a really good job. A week before I was to be there, he called to tell me he was leaving. The official announcement would come two days prior to my arrival. He had worked really hard, and unbelievably neat things were taking place. When I show up, managers and others are grieving. I changed the workshop agenda and did the workshop on what can be done to make sure all the positive work sticks.

A key indicator of when the culture is going to stick is coworkers saying to coworkers, "This is how we do it here." The culture is safe when it is the organization's way of doing things and not dependent on who is in senior leadership. That's when you know you've really created that culture of ownership.

Coworkers also drive retention. Mark Faulkner, currently the CEO and president of Baptist Health Care, headquartered in Pensacola, Florida, told me back when he was working with me at Baptist as the administrator of Jay Hospital, "I wake up every morning figuring out how to retain the people who are working here." We're all chief retention officers. And I don't mean just the leaders. I mean everyone, because not only do people leave their boss, they leave their coworker.

The best thing we all can do is create that culture where people not only want to work there themselves, but also want to tell other people, "You should work here too." People in healthcare talk. They know the best places to work and the best people to work for.

If you create the right culture, the right culture keeps perpetuating the right culture…and that culture keeps retaining employees.

CHAPTER 22

Contempt Prior to Investigation

There are times when we all need to say, "I'm sorry." We make mistakes sometimes, or forget to connect the dots, or get caught up in circumstances that make us late for meetings. Many times, things happen that are beyond our control. As much as we wish we could control them, we just can't. When these things happen—and they do happen to us all—it means a lot when others give us the benefit of the doubt. And as much as possible, we need to do the same for them.

One time I had a meeting scheduled with Dr. Floyd Loop. He was instrumental in the Cleveland Clinic's being what it is today. Dr. Loop was always good about meeting with me when I was on campus, but this time it didn't happen. He didn't show up at the scheduled time, and I didn't know exactly what happened. He canceled and I flew back to Pensacola, Florida.

That night I received an email from Dr. Loop. He apologized for not meeting with me. He shared that his best friend was dying. He had spent the last six and a half hours in the hospital room holding his friend's hand. Dr. Loop wrote to me, "I so apologize for missing our meeting; sometimes life just does that." And it made such an impact on me when he wrote this and connected.

Here is where we see the benefit of reputation. I was never angry with Dr. Loop, only concerned. His reputation was impeccable. I had always found him to be a man of his word, fair and trustworthy. If I had not had such trust in Dr. Loop, I may have thought he was blowing me off, and worse, I could have shared my sentiments with others prior to knowing the whole story.

Herbert Spencer wrote, "There is a principle which is a bar against all information, which is proof against all argument and which cannot fail to keep a man in everlasting ignorance. This principle is contempt prior to investigation." Contempt prior to investigation happens often in the workplace. In stressful and hurried environments, it's even more prevalent.

It may look something like this: Without knowing all the facts, an employee may think a leader has done something wrong. They may approach the leader in a forceful or upset way that shows the "contempt" Herbert Spencer wrote about. They might send an accusatory email. Or it might be the other way around. Maybe the leader makes an incorrect assumption about an employee and approaches that individual from a place of anger.

The person who shows contempt prior to investigation might say hurtful things that are hard to take back. These statements can cause real damage to the relationship. What happens next is the target of the contempt gets defensive. They feel attacked and are probably not inclined to help fix the problem.

We need to have the emotional maturity to pause before coming to a conclusion and/or taking action before we know the whole story. And we need to be careful with our words. It is too easy to assume the worst and say things we will later regret. How we approach a situation is everything. Imagine if we just opened by saying, "I could be wrong, but this is my perception. Could you please help me understand what happened?" When we do this, we'll most likely find what we assumed is incorrect. We will have set a different tone for the conversation and paved the way for a healthy dialogue. We'll have put the focus back on fixing the problem at hand.

There's another side of the story as well. Let's look at the other side of the "contempt prior to investigation" issue. When we do a good job of narrating why we do what we do—especially when we have to make decisions that might upset people—we can prevent people from having to "investigate." What we need to do is head the contempt off at the pass. And when we do mess up, we need to say we're sorry.

Good Communication Helps Others NOT Assume the Worst.

I received a call from a CEO who was concerned about some negative pushback he was receiving. They had let a number of people go, and the workforce was very upset. How could they be building a new building and not have enough money to keep all the workforce? He explained to me that the current projects being built were being built with borrowed funds and to not finish them would be a financial disaster. The expansions would help the organization when the projects were completed. What had happened was that reimbursement for some of their services had decreased more than anticipated. New technology meant that procedures that had required hospital stays now were done outpatient. To maintain the current bond rating (the bond rating impacts the interest rate paid), he shared that he needed to move quickly and in hindsight realized the communication they did was not enough. This had a negative impact on the organization. We discussed what steps he could take. I feel he knew what needed to take place but asked me to get a second opinion.

Now, do any of us like reductions of force? Absolutely not. But they sometimes happen, and they will continue to happen at times.

Over several days and nights, the CEO met in town halls with all the staff. He said, "I apologize. I know I moved quickly. I know this hurts a lot of us because these were people we had worked with for a long time. Let me go back now and walk you through the thought process of how this happened and why it moved so quickly."

He scheduled a series of sessions with all staff. At each session, the group was divided into small tables and they asked, "If this happens again, which it might, how can we do a better job of connecting the dots and explaining it?" He also said, "Here is what I have learned." After the sessions, people still felt bad about the reduction in force, but they understood it better. And they were now part of the communication in the future after attending the sessions.

One of the CEOs I respect tremendously called me because his employee engagement had just bottomed out. He had been working for years to build up employee engagement, not because of the numbers, but because of what it represented. I've often said to healthcare people, metrics are nice to tally, but people don't get excited about the metric—they get excited about what the metric means.

So we talked. He was disappointed in himself. He shared that things were moving so fast with COVID-19, and while he did his best to communicate, at times rumors moved more quickly than truth. He wasn't sure what to do, what to stop doing, how to protect people, and so on. He asked, "What should I do?"

I responded, "Well, what are your thoughts?" He gave me his thoughts, I reinforced what he was already thinking, and added a few suggestions. He had come up with a good plan on his own but it helps to reach out for feedback before moving forward.

So this CEO decided to meet with his staff (some virtually because of the situation). He apologized, then explained, "I could have communicated better. I hear you loud and clear. I certainly wish I would have said this earlier, but let me walk through the timeline of what happened."

When he finished talking, he created a rapid response task force to create tools and techniques so that when something unexpected happens this quickly in the future it can be handled better. Immediately, people got it. People want their boss to be successful. They want the leadership team to do well, because if they don't do well, the rest of the organization doesn't do well.

When we say we're sorry, it's not just about showing people that we care. It's also about helping others understand that we're all human. We all make mistakes. None of us know it all. We all need to give each other grace. When we acknowledge these things and show our vulnerability, we create a real sense of human connection.

CHAPTER 23

Turning Obstacles Into Opportunities

I've noticed over the years that people in healthcare are so resilient. I was with a cardiovascular surgeon one day, and he got a phone call from a patient he had operated on 30 years ago. It was the patient's birthday, and he was reaching out to the surgeon to thank him for his life. He said that without the operation, he would not be alive today.

After the phone call, the cardiovascular surgeon explained to me that this had been a case where during surgery, it became obvious the patient would not live unless something changed. Knowing this, he tried a different technique he'd never tried before. It was something he thought would work, but he had never done it. But at the time, he knew if he didn't try something out of the ordinary what the outcome would be. He tweaked the procedure and ended up saving this man's life. It turned out to be a procedure that's now used in hospitals across the country.

This surgeon used his creativity. An obstacle he faced became an opportunity. I've seen that often when I look at people in healthcare—the creativity is just amazing.

People also have their own personal obstacles that provide opportunities. I remember a story I heard in a hospital: A young lady had ovarian cancer, and she was going in for major surgery. She was terrified she was going to die. A nurse heard about her and went and sat with her. One of the things the nurse said to her was, "I had this exact same procedure you're having six years ago." So what this young lady heard was that this nurse had the same procedure six years ago, but she's sitting here now, which connected the dots that she's not going to die. This nurse took what was an obstacle for her at one time and turned it into an opportunity to help other people.

Tara Blackwell lives in the Pensacola area. She was a great high school athlete and went to Troy University on a softball scholarship. One day after a practice on an away trip with her team, she did a backflip, but landed wrong and suffered a cervical spinal cord injury, fracturing her fifth and sixth vertebrae. She was paralyzed. She has limited use of her body from her shoulders down with some hand movement. Tara now runs an adaptive rehabilitation center called The Seven Project, which serves those living with physical disabilities, focusing on day-to-day quality-of-life enhancement through fitness, nutrition, and support. Not only did Tara take an obstacle and make it an opportunity, but she created an opportunity for other people. Tara recently posted a quote I love on Instagram: "Imagine the best version of yourself and show up every day as her."

We all have our own individual obstacles we face in life and sometimes it takes somebody who's been through it to help somebody else. I didn't realize at times that some obstacles I faced were going to be opportunities, but they did become those. Many of you who have heard me speak know I have a hearing impairment. I'm deaf in my right ear and hear a little bit in my left ear. What you might not know is that at one time, my right ear was my better ear, and my left ear was worse. Now it's the opposite. This has always been a struggle for me. If you don't hear, you don't know what you're missing because you can't hear it.

But let me explain what a great opportunity being hearing impaired has been for me. One, I've always had to really focus on listening because it's so hard to hear. I have to look at people's lips very closely to understand what they are saying, so I'm very focused on them. The benefit of this is people feel really good talking to somebody who's paying so much attention to what they're saying and looking right at them. So even though I don't hear well, I believe I'm a very good listener. In fact, people have tested me and I can almost repeat back everything they said to me verbatim, because I've had to train myself to be such a still listener. An obstacle, a hearing impairment, ended up being a benefit to me and an opportunity to become a better listener.

I also had a speech impediment. Until I was five years old, my mother was the only person who could interpret what I was saying. She understood when I said "bulk," B-U-L-K, that meant "milk."

When I went to kindergarten, I was immediately put into speech class. Once a week, a speech pathologist would come to the classroom and get me, and we'd walk to the speech pathology room. Speech pathologists have a difficult job because they're asking people to repeat words over and over again. They are great motivators who inspire people to keep trying even though they may be uncomfortable and frustrated with the repetition and sense of failure.

Now, if you think about it, that's what leadership is. Leadership many times is doing something we're extremely uncomfortable with over and over again until we're comfortable doing it. I really believe that those years of speech therapy helped me learn to stick with things even when they're difficult because I was programmed early on that I had to do difficult things and be uncomfortable in order to get the desired outcome. So a speech impediment became something very positive for me.

Today, I still often mispronounce words. I've figured out that when I mispronounce a word, it's best to keep right on going. I know that when I talk sometimes I completely mess up a word. It makes sense in my brain, but somehow between my brain and my mouth there's a disconnect, and it comes out different than I had planned. I've talked to so many intelligent people over the years, and I've watched their faces when I've mispronounced a word and kept talking. I can almost see them thinking, *Wow, he's smart. I've never heard that word before.* Well, they've never heard it because there is no such word!

Good humor can also be the result of an obstacle becoming an opportunity. I've also found that other people take that the same way, and we can all learn from this attitude.

CHAPTER 24

It's Better to Be Interested Than Interesting

Many of us need to get better at being *interested*, not *interesting*. This is true in all industries but it's especially true in healthcare. It's pretty obvious that the more interested we are in patients the better we are at treating them. Asking good questions and really paying attention to the answers leads to good diagnoses and care plans.

What we may not always realize is the same holds true for leaders. Being interested in other people (rather than trying to be interesting to them) engages them, gets them to open up, and creates authentic connections. It gets us beyond arm's length and creates the kind of relationships with employees that inspire them to do their best work.

Now when I say this, I'm not implying that leaders are self-involved or ego-driven. It's just that it's natural to want to hear our own voices and tell our own stories. A lot of this has to do with the signals we get all our lives. We are taught that to be leaders we need to come across as experts, always sharing advice and giving feedback.

Being interested in and listening to others isn't always emphasized. But it's what gets results.

During my years of traveling, I would turn on the TV when I got into a hotel room. I would just flip on these shows that required little thinking to let my mind relax for a while, and one was called *Blind Date*. It's not on anymore. There are probably reasons they took it off the air, but I found it interesting. The show introduced two people and had them go on a date. They showed the date on TV, and the viewer would watch them interact.

Then at the end of the show, they would ask each person, "Based on the experience you just had, would you go out with this person again?" And it was pretty interesting to see how sometimes one person would say yes and one person would say no. I started wondering, *What is the difference? Why would one person say yes but the other person say no?* And it seemed to come down to this: Those individuals who were interested in the other person tended to be the ones the other person would like to see again. But for those people who were busy being interesting, the blind date would say, "No, they seem too self-oriented."

I started thinking about this in the context of healthcare. Are we *interested* or *interesting?* Most of healthcare is demonstrating interest. Physicians are experts in this. When they interact with the patient, they show interest in how the patient is feeling, how medication is working, and so forth. Interested physicians are good physicians.

Also, being interested creates a much better patient experience. When we do a pre-call for someone before they come in for an appointment, we're really interested in making sure they're going to be prepared for it. When we call, text, or email a patient after they leave the hospital or clinic to make sure they are okay, we're interested. Much of the pre- and post-appointment communication is online now, but we can still explain why we're contacting them. Instead of just sending a patient an online form to fill out before a doctor's appointment, why not include a paragraph that reads, "We're sending this form for you to complete in advance because we want you to be prepared for your appointment and we want to be prepared as well. We want to ensure that we know all your concerns before your arrival so you can get the very best care possible."

I think when we meet people it's our natural instinct to try to be interesting, as we think that's what makes people like us. We need to shift our mindset to the understanding that people will like us more if we show interest in THEM rather than talking about ourselves. One way to do this is to be prepared with a few questions that work across a lot of different scenarios. I heard a story once about a person who was seated at the table with the brand new CEO of his company, a great opportunity for sure. He resisted the urge to try to impress the CEO with great stories about himself, but instead turned to him and said, "So, how did you get your start?" The CEO went on to tell him an incredible story. It broke the tension and created a great bond between the two.

Think about people you've met, leaders you've worked with, friends you've had. You're probably not as attracted to those who talk more about themselves and are less interested in listening to you. In my work with universities, one of the common questions I get is about interviews. I say, "What you want is for the interviewer to talk more than you do. If they talk more than you do, you're going to have a pretty good chance of getting that job. The interviewer will enjoy the interview if you focus more on being interested than on being interesting. Human beings have a natural tendency to enjoy talking to someone who is interested in them."

This is why most of us need to get better at self-awareness *and* situational awareness. Both skills help us notice when we are focusing too much on ourselves and need to redirect our focus to others.

All of this applies to leadership as well. Many of the tools and tactics we use are around showing that we are interested.

Some Tactics That Show Employees You're Interested

Leader rounding. Essentially, when we talk about rounding, we're talking about a formalized way of being *interested* in staff members. We commit to devoting a certain amount of time each week to meeting with employees and asking a set of questions:

First we ask a question aimed at building our relationship with that employee. For example, "How is your daughter doing in college?" "How was your vacation?" "Is your mother doing better now?"

Then we ask other questions related to the job:

"What is working well today?"

"Do you have everything you need to do your job?"

"Are there any individuals I should be recognizing?"

"Is there anything we can do better?"

By asking all of these questions—and by taking action based on their answers—we are showing that we are truly interested in making their employee experience better. And it works. We find over and over that regular leader rounding is one of the most powerful things we can do to create employee satisfaction.

Anything we can do to get to know people better can help us be genuinely interested in them. It reminds me of something I learned from Susan Keane Baker, a speaker and author I really enjoy. She has terrific ideas on how to better connect with patients and employees. She tells a wonderful story about how on a neuro ICU unit at New York-Presbyterian/Columbia new colleagues were invited to bring something of value with them to a morning huddle as kind of a "get-to-know-you" tactic. Gregory, a new registered nurse, brought in his marine uniform. I can only imagine how many connections were made after he shared that and how interested people were in getting to know him!

If you have never rounded before, it can be uncomfortable and even a little scary. But we see over and over that regular leader rounding is one of the most powerful things we can do to engage employees and keep them happy. And the good news is, the more we do it, the easier it will become.

Duncan Finlay, MD, is a good example of someone who discovered the power of leader rounding. He was a pulmonologist at Sarasota Memorial Hospital in Sarasota, Florida. He was the chief medical officer, and the CEO there took a new job. The board asked Dr. Finlay to fill the CEO role until they found a permanent CEO.

Dr. Finlay asked me to round with him. He said he'd rounded as a doctor, but he had never rounded as a CEO. I remember the first time we rounded, we saw two ladies reading a sign in the hallway outside a waiting area. Obviously they had a family member or friend in the hospital. I approached them and said, "My name is Quint Studer. I'm here working with the hospital, and this is Duncan Finlay. He's the president of the hospital. Do you have someone here?" And they said, "Oh yes, our brother is a patient here." I asked them what they thought of his care and they responded, "The care is wonderful." I could see Dr. Finlay relax when he heard they were pleased with their brother's care.

I then said, "Dr. Finlay loves to reward and recognize staff for providing excellent care to patients. Is there anyone in particular you would like him to reward and recognize?" They didn't know people by name, but they were able to describe a few people on the unit we could recognize. Dr. Finlay is a quick learner. He said, "While your brother is here, if you see any other people you would like recognized, please write their names down and either give them to the unit secretary or bring them down to my office." Then Dr. Finlay told them where his office was and he chatted with them for a bit—he was a natural relationship-builder. After a very brief experience, Dr. Finlay got it.

He called a department manager meeting that afternoon, and he said to everyone, "We need to own the hallways. We need to make sure that every time we see someone in the hallway, we create a conversation. We need to find out why they're there, where they're going, how we can help them, and whom we can recognize." Through his leadership, Sarasota Memorial became a real leader in healthcare, which continues today.

At first, we may be scared to make these connections. We are fearful of what people might say, and fearful that we can't meet their requests. But as leaders, being close to employees and patients gives us a real chance to see how we *can* help. It also gives us a chance to fill our own emotional bank account. It's what makes the job so incredibly fulfilling. Showing up is everything, even if you are scared.

Be honest about what you can and can't do. Even when you have to say, "I'm sorry, I can't make that happen"—and explain why—people will appreciate your transparency. Authentic interactions with people build trust and fill emotional bank accounts. Leader rounding helps you build these kinds of connections. It lets people know you care. Feeling like they have been heard can go a long way. Just being available for conversations is an opportunity to fix a lot of things.

Training and professional development. When we provide training and professional development, we are helping them get better at what they do and advance in their organization and career. Most people really care about professional development. A Gallup survey found that 87 percent of millennials said professional or career growth and development are important to them.[1] Just be sure to narrate, "I care about your professional development," so they'll know you are interested in them and want the best for them. And be sure to check in and see how it's going. Ask, "Are there new things you want to learn? Anything you are struggling with?"

Great leaders make training and development a priority. I did some training at the Cleveland Clinic years ago. The late Dr. Floyd D. Loop was CEO at the time, and he was present during the entire session. I remember hearing physicians say this is when they knew the training was really important to the organization. Over the years, I have made the statement that one can evaluate a person's and/or organization's values by their commitment to providing the workforce with training and development.

Regular one-on-one meetings. As with professional development, regular performance and feedback meetings show employees we want to help them become better and better. The kind of meetings I'm talking about here go beyond the "official" annual performance review. I am talking about meeting with employees at least once a quarter to engage in goal-setting, provide solid feedback, and in general let them know how much you value them. When we hold these one-on-one meetings, we are making time to say, "I am interested in you, I care about you, and I want to set you up to succeed."

Also, it's important to hold 30- and 90-day meetings with recent hires. Basically, this means scheduling a time to sit down one-on-one with a new employee and ask key questions to help them alleviate anxiety, find out what they need, and work through any difficulties they may be having. We're saying, "We're interested to see how you're adjusting to your new job." As you learned in Chapter 13, 30- and 90-day meetings are incredibly valuable in helping us retain new employees.

Reward and recognition. An entire chapter is devoted to this one (See Chapter 15). Essentially, when we reward and recognize employees—not just employees but also physicians and leaders at all levels—we are showing them that we see all the good things they are doing. We're not just interested; we're grateful.

A focus on listening. Learn to be a better listener and teach your team, too. Being a great listener is a fundamental part of being a great communicator, and a vital part of showing others you're interested. You, your leaders, and your whole team can benefit from learning to be better listeners. Leonard H. Friedman is a professor in the Department of Health Policy and Management at George Washington University and is a director of the Executive Master of Health Administration (MHA@GW) program. As a professor, he's always looking for new ideas to teach foundational skills to students. He shared a great exercise:

> I use a listening exercise that I learned from someone I met while at Oregon State University, Paul Axtell. Paul taught me a technique to improve the quality of conversations. The idea here is that all human relationships are created via a series of conversations. At the heart of all conversations is the ability to listen to one another. I pair up students in groups of two and provide everyone with a series of questions, including things like, *What was your favorite childhood memory? When was a time that you made a difference? Why did you decide to enter the profession of healthcare management?* The rule is that each person must be allowed to speak uninterrupted on the agreed-upon topic for three minutes. After the three minutes has elapsed, we switch roles. The idea here is to give everyone the experience of being heard and allowed to speak without the other person taking over the conversation.

Being interested works well with all people. It completely changes the way they see you. And it takes a lot of pressure off—once you realize that you don't have to keep trying to prove you're the smartest person in the room, it's amazing how much you'll enjoy connecting with the people around you, and how much you'll learn in the process.

Consider the popular saying "People don't care how much you know until they know how much you care." *Interested* shows caring. And caring creates high-performing organizations.

As we implement new tactics to become more interested and caring, one thing we have on our side is the fact that we are lifelong learners. Healthcare is a vocation in which learning and adjusting to change is a constant process. What most healthcare people have in common is a deep desire to learn. We are so driven to do a good job, to be helpful and useful, that underneath the discomfort we may feel, we are grateful for opportunities to learn and grow. And the more we do new things, the easier they become.

When we can see the impact of the actions we take, it connects to values. Once they are part of our values, we cannot *not* do what is best for those we work with and care for.

CHAPTER 25

Track Yourself

One of my issues is I talk way too much. In fact, I was born talking. All my relatives would complain and say to my mother, "Doesn't that kid ever shut up?" My mother thinks it's funny that something people complained about ended up being beneficial. My love for talking has allowed me to provide for my parents and relatives. Unfortunately, I sometimes talk *too much*. When I have an idea, I don't have the self-restraint to be quiet.

Have you ever watched the show *Welcome Back, Kotter?* I'm the Horshack character. Something I've done over the years is to make a checkmark every time I talk in meetings. Every time I speak, I put a little mark on a paper. That helps me monitor how much I am speaking. I might even put a mark when other people in the room are speaking. It's not that I'm evaluating their speaking, but I want to balance the amount of my own talking out with the rest of the group.

In fact, sometimes I even write a little note to myself and I use the initials "KMBMS." And if you're wondering what that stands for, it's "Keep my big mouth shut." I want to be a better listener, so this is a chance to break a bad habit. It's a way for me to see that I'm dominating the conversation by overtalking and not giving other people a chance.

There is real power in writing things down. Let's say you have an employee who seems to come in late to work quite a bit. Until you actually start documenting the occurrences, you can't tell if the tardiness problem is real or just an impression you have. Sometimes, our mind plays tricks on us.

The same holds true in our personal lives. Tracking helps us succeed in goals we really want to work on. Think about how we use calorie counters and fitness trackers to monitor our food intake and exercise. Food journals are another great example. Studies show that those who keep food records tend to lose more weight than those who don't.

Why does tracking work so well? Partly it's because it provides a true picture of what's happening. Data doesn't lie. You might have the impression that you're not eating much throughout the day, but when you write down every bite you take, you might come to see you really are snacking too much.

Also, tracking holds you accountable to yourself. You can better resist the urge to cheat if you see your actions there in black and white. It will also help you identify patterns. Are there certain times of the day when you eat more? Are there certain types of meetings where you talk more? Because of the accountability factor, tracking is a great tool to help you set and celebrate goals.

It's not just good for stopping things, either. It can help you make sure you are doing the things you intend to do. In the same way we track ourselves to break a bad habit, we can track ourselves to create the kind of life we want to create. We can figure out what we are doing that keeps us away from the things we enjoy. In a very real way, it gives us some time back.

Here is a technique I picked up when I was in behavioral health that can help you not move away from what you enjoy. When people would come into treatment, they would be asked, "What do you love?" And people would talk about how they love fishing or how they love cooking. They love being with their family. They love traveling. And then they were asked, "When was the last time you did that?" And they'd realize, even though they said they loved it, they hadn't done it in a while. Of course, the reason they hadn't done it in a while is because their addiction took them away from doing a lot of things they loved.

Now, we all have challenges with our balance of life. Or rather, we have challenges with our *blending* of life, if you don't like the word *balance*. How do we blend all our activities? I think one of the things that's nice to do is just take time to answer the question, "What are the things you really enjoy?" Write down your answers. And then over the next couple of weeks or months, just track when you do those things. I think if you are like me, it will help you start to realize, "These are some things I really enjoy doing, but I'm just not doing them right now. Or I'm not doing them often enough."

When we see on paper what we're doing that we don't want to do—and we're not doing what we *do* want to do—it can really inspire us to make some changes. We can stop doing things that aren't productive and start doing things we really want to do. This is how we start to take back our most valuable commodity: our time.

Ultimately, we are responsible for living the life we want to live. It is up to us to determine how we can best serve others and live up to our calling. No one else can do it for us. We need to own our own well-being. Self-monitoring helps us do that. Tracking ourselves is a powerful tool—one that's life-changing when we make the effort to do it regularly.

CHAPTER 26

Telehealth: Marrying Technology and the Human Connection

I first saw the potential of telehealth back in 2011 when I was invited to speak in China on a ten-day tour by the Chinese Hospital Association. I was shown a room that looked like an air traffic control center in which patients were being seen via video. In this situation, the person was in an exam room with a healthcare provider. They were getting access to expertise not available where they lived.

Then, in 2016, I presented at a venture capital conference on healthcare investments. There were four hour-long sessions running from 8:00 a.m. to 12:00 p.m. The room was packed. It was during the election campaign of Hillary Clinton and Donald Trump, so the election was a hot topic. The first presentation was by Bobby Jindal, former governor of Louisiana, and James Carville, a political consultant. The second presentation was by Patrick J. Kennedy on the issue of opiate use and addiction. Then there was a break.

My first thought was very few in the audience would be coming back after the break. I was presenting next and then there was a panel. To my surprise, the room stayed packed. For a moment, I thought I must be a bigger draw than expected. But after my presentation, I found out it wasn't me who had brought people back. The organizers knew they needed a big closer, so they had scheduled a panel to discuss the future of telehealth.

Fast forward to the pandemic. In early March of 2020, I was teaching at George Washington University. They have an outstanding faculty. In a discussion with a faculty member, the topic of telehealth came up along with reimbursement for this method of care delivery. The rest is history.

My point is that we've had the technology and the know-how for quite some time, but the pandemic accelerated the delivery of virtual care. Being on the board for two healthcare providers, I had a good seat to view the implementation of virtual care. It's not that telehealth hadn't been advancing. It had. It's that the pandemic accelerated progress exponentially.

Telehealth provides such a wonderful opportunity to improve access for patients. A friend's wife has arthritis and going to see her physician isn't easy. At her age, she was apprehensive about how a virtual visit would work. To the credit of her doctor, the first virtual visit went great. Afterward, she told her husband that she felt she preferred to have the virtual visits from now on unless it was necessary to actually go into the doctor's office.

In the area of behavioral medicine, telemedicine has been provided in the past, particularly in rural areas. But the pandemic led to expanded use. Without access to virtual meetings, the toll on people in recovery would have been even worse.

My curiosity led me to learn more about telehealth and how providers were helping caregivers adapt. As with any change, there are
"first movers." I reached out to former colleagues of mine, Dan Smith,
MD, and Stephen Beeson, MD. Both shared videos they had made, as
well as written articles with suggested approaches. My friends at Dea-
coness Midtown Hospital in Evansville, Indiana, invited me to join a
virtual session to discuss best practices and lessons learned. My search
has led me to speak with many people on this topic. Again, this is a
time of learning.

I agree with the great majority of tips I received. However, there
are a few areas I have questions about (not that I am necessarily right,
but just wondering). One that comes to mind—and it showed up
quite a bit in my search—is a suggestion to providers to always look at
the camera. I thought about how when I'm at my doctor's office, they
usually look at me while we're talking. However, at times they don't,
and when they handle those times the right way, it's fine.

My long-time primary care specialist was Dr. Anita Westafer. I am
still getting over her retirement. When we were together, there were
times she would say, "Let me look that up." She would then focus on
the computer screen to pull up past results and other pertinent information. When she didn't look at me, I understood why. My suggestion since then to providers holding a telehealth visit is not only is it
okay, but it may also help the patient feel better to have the provider
say, "Let me pull this up," or, "Let's look at this." In most instances,
narrating care makes a very positive difference.

The leaders at a medical group noticed that a physician they all
like, and feel is a very good physician, had poor patient experience
results. In observing the physician, it was noticed that he was very
focused on documenting everything he heard from the patient in their
medical record. This meant his eye contact with the patient wasn't
good. My experience is that at times when we make suggestions, a
provider will say, "If I do what you advise, it will take more time."

So, if we said to the physician, "You need to have better eye contact," we may hear, "If I do, my productivity will go down. What do you want? Better patient experience or better productivity?" (Others may not have ever had this experience.)

Here is what happened. The advice to the physician was, "Keep doing exactly what you are doing. Just add an explanation." In other words, say to the patient, "While you are speaking, I want to capture it in your medical record. This means we won't have eye contact. This isn't because I don't want to have eye contact; it is due to my goal to make sure I capture everything in your medical record so I can provide you with great care." He may have tweaked this language, of course. The point is that by adding this brief explanation, his patient experience skyrocketed, and productivity stayed strong. Often, it isn't the behavior that results in less-than-desired outcomes; it is the lack of explanation for the behavior. It is the *why*. This tactic should also work when consulting with patients in a telehealth capacity.

My search led me to Swati Mehta, MD, FACP. I love her work in "Make Your Virtual Visit R.E.A.L." As I studied her work, I contacted her. Since then, we have had many conversations on her learnings and those of others. Her framework for holding impactful virtual visits centers on the acronym "R.E.A.L."

Patients can have some anxiety about virtual visits. At every point in the interaction, Dr. Mehta provides a list of questions to ask yourself, helpful phrases to say, and actions to take. She gives lots of helpful reminders to do the little things that make the patient more comfortable. Here is just a brief overview:

Ready. In this step, the clinician introduces themselves, does an audiovisual check, and inquires about any family members who might be included in the visit.

Establish Agenda and Expectations. They discuss the patient's concerns. The clinician may address the "looking away from the camera" issue by saying something like, "I have your medical record pulled up. If you see me looking away/down, it's because I am checking your blood work results, etc."

Authentic Connection. The clinician smiles, leans in, looks at the camera for "direct eye contact," asks questions to make a personal connection, and responds to patient anxiety with statements like, "I am so sorry you had to go through that."

Lay Out Plans and Next Steps. Clinician wraps up, focusing on simplicity and comprehension. They make it clear what they will do and what the patient will do.

Another great source of information on this subject is Tom Dahlborg. He is an industry voice for relationship-centered compassionate care and the author of the wonderful book *From Heart to Head & Back Again…a Journey through the Healthcare System.*

Tom says technology needs to be recognized as a tool, not as a solution. You still have to leverage a number of different things to ensure that leveraging technology would work. This includes mindfulness, empathy, and maintaining the intention to recognize and honor the emotions of others. At the end of the day, it's all about that authentic relationship.

Technology can be incredibly scary. Tom shared this story about a nursing home. With the pandemic, families were not being let in, so of course the residents were lonely. Studies have shown that loneliness is more dangerous than smoking, so by itself it is an incredible health challenge. Many of these wonderful organizations and caring people were trying to leverage technology to help alleviate the loneliness. This nursing home was one of them.

Tom shared that when the facility tried to use iPads to connect residents with family, it was actually causing more stress than the loneliness. The residents weren't brought up with that type of technology so they were uncomfortable trying to use it. There was no time allotted and no system created to help educate them, to help them understand, and to walk them through the process. This would have gone a long way toward helping this effort be successful.

His point was that we need to learn to walk side by side with this technology. It's going to be a bridge between the provider and the patient, but we need to keep the human factor in mind as we implement it.

Sometimes as providers we are focused on what we need to do. We don't always look through the lens of the patient and family, especially the most vulnerable populations. Tom says that for telehealth to really take hold, we will have to build the system with the patient in mind. How will we keep this human connection that we all need so badly—not just the patient but also the provider?

We have to make sure we're not so focused on getting information to leverage technology to improve care that we forget the compassion and the love and the empathy and the fear that the patient is going through. The human factor is what fuels our calling as healthcare providers.

David Callecod, former president and CEO of Lafayette General Health System, says they worked very hard to ask themselves, *How do we create the same experience, the same sense of culture, virtually?* He adds that others need to ask this question as well. For instance, in Lafayette General's case, they focus on reducing patient anxiety via AIDET®—an acronym that stands for Acknowledge, Introduce, Duration, Explanation, and Thank You. (NOTE: See Chapter 19 for more information on AIDET.) The idea is to give providers key words to apply the same level of great care to virtual visits.

Telehealth is a new door we just opened, and if done well, it can be amazing. The pandemic created a situation where many could not see providers, and virtual visits were great options. When one door closes, one opens, but it's hell in the hallways for a while. Right now, we may be in the hallway stage, with everyone adjusting. For a while, we may need to overexplain and overcompensate. That's okay. Like any change, it takes time to be comfortable. Telehealth can make access to care better for many…and with the right tools and development in place, along with fair reimbursement, it can improve the lives of providers as well.

CHAPTER 27

Storytelling Helps People Connect to the Difference They Make

Healthcare people make a huge difference in the lives of others. Often they don't even realize the impact they make. Yet knowing that we do make a difference is what feeds and strengthens self-motivation and keeps us doing our best work when times get tough. This is why it is so important that we remind healthcare workers of this truth again and again. People need to hear that they make a difference.

In my first book, *Hardwiring Excellence*, I wrote about the huge impact my high school soccer coach had on me. His coaching style taught me the power of starting with the positive. Here is the excerpt:

> Later, when I went to high school, I decided to play soccer because it was the only sport where they didn't cut anybody. My soccer coach Mr. King had a way of correcting me without destroying me. He would come up to me and say, "Quint, way to hustle! Way to get to that ball!" Then, almost as an afterthought, he'd add,

"Next time, *let's put the foot out*. But hey, you got there! Way to go!"

You know how I felt? Pretty good. I had hustled. I had gotten there. And the next time, you better believe that I remembered to put my foot out. What if he had said, "Quint! What's the matter with you? What good does it do for you to run all that way if you don't kick the ball? Sit down now so I can put somebody else in."

I might have run a little slower the next time to make sure I didn't get yelled at for missing the ball. Coach King taught me to go for the ball. If we only hear about what we can't do, it seems easier to give up. Many of us do. In fact, of the people who leave their jobs at a healthcare organization, a great many leave within the first 90 days. About 27 percent of all employees who leave do so during this early period of employment. They don't leave to go work in some other industry. They just give up on their current healthcare employer and try another one. I believe this is because they hear too much about what they can't do instead of what they can do.[1]

I am asked by people if I ever saw Coach King after high school to say thank you. The answer is yes. To tell that story, I need to tell the story of Cam Underhill.

She left us way too young, passing away from breast cancer. She worked in Easley, South Carolina, at a hospital called Baptist Easley. She would come to Studer Group's Taking You and Your Organization to the Next Level (TYYO) conferences and was always so engaged. She was the fire starter among all fire starters. In fact, when she passed away, the hospital created an area where all the employees come into the hospital and there's a fire there: a constant fire there to represent Cam.

Every organization has Cam Underhills. Healthcare is filled with passionate people doing their best to make life better for others.

The hospital Cam worked for did great leadership development training. At the one I attended, many physicians and board members were present. Cam asked me to tell the Coach King story as part of my presentation. So I did. As I closed with this story, Cam brought Coach King up on stage. She had actually flown him in from Chicago into the Carolinas so he could walk out onstage, and I could talk to him and thank him.

These are the things that we sometimes don't get to do. Sometimes people don't know they have made such a difference in our lives. Coach King was certainly not aware of his impact. In many situations, healthcare workers are not aware of the tremendous difference they make.

Also in *Hardwiring Excellence*, I have a section in the Conclusion called "Brian's Story" where I tell the story about my nephew. In 1995, at 19 years old, he was killed in a car wreck. Four years later, I spoke at Christ Hospital on the South Side of Chicago in Oak Lawn, the hospital he was taken to and where he was declared dead. They didn't know about Brian's death, but I shared the story and thanked them for the care they gave Brian when he was in their hospital.

Later, I got a note from the emergency room nurse telling me how she always thought about my family around the holidays. Now, she would not have heard that thank you if I hadn't come there to speak, because when it happened, the family was so torn and grieving over the loss of their 19-year-old son. Sometimes we want to say thanks. It's just that too many things are going on.

My message here is don't underestimate the difference you make. Don't think that you're not making a difference because maybe a person doesn't tell you, doesn't show you, or doesn't write you. Now, I know healthcare workers don't do what they do for the accolades.

They don't do it for a thank-you note. They don't do it for a plaque. They do it because their DNA has called them to be helpful and useful.

Here is one of my favorite stories I've heard over the years. A nurse went to her daughter's kindergarten open house. She sat down at the daughter's desk, and the woman next to her said, "I have a picture of you in my wallet." At first, the woman was thinking, *Whoa, what do we have here?*

And then the mom said, "My daughter was born prematurely." She was referring to the daughter who was now in kindergarten. The mom added, "We did not know if she was going to live. I so wanted a picture, and they took a picture of her in the incubator for me. You were the nurse with your hands in the incubator holding my baby." And she showed the nurse that picture.

Now, this nurse would have never known that was the type of impact she had when she went to help that mom get a picture of her baby. But because she happened to be sitting next to her at a kindergarten open house, she found out. These kinds of stories are so remarkable to me.

In the book *A Culture of High Performance*, I include a story from a lady who lost her son. She was at a Harris Teeter supermarket and saw the nurse who was there when her son was brought to the ED. In her letter, she describes their encounter and how healing it was:

A Word of Gratitude

The following words, written by Wendy Mayo on her blog after the loss of her son Zack, reveal the impact a healthcare professional can have on someone's life:

I was standing in the check-out line at Harris Teeter when I saw her. Her face was familiar but I could not be certain. She and three girls stood in the line next to me. I looked again, trying not to be obvious, but trying harder to remember. Then I heard her speak to one of the girls.

And I knew. **Her voice.** And I remembered and I swallowed hard. Swallowing down the memory of that day.

That day in June.

She was the voice that called out to us in the Emergency Room.

She was the voice that was commanding, yet kind.

She was the voice that told us our 11-year-old son had no cardiac activity.

She was the voice that ushered us to a small room.

She was the voice that stayed late into the night to care for our family needs in the beginning of our darkest hours.

She was the voice of compassion.

Her name I could not remember. But I did remember her voice....

I hurried to pay—hoping I could leave before her. Instead I followed her out of the store—purposely keeping distance between us. Afraid she would recognize me? Purposely avoiding her? Purposely avoiding the still raw emotions from that day nearly two and a half years ago....

Groceries loaded in my car, I wanted to jump in and speed away. But a voice inside me urged. **Find her.**

Silent gratitude isn't much use to anyone.
—G.B. Stern

And I found myself across a dark parking lot standing face to face with the voice who was loading groceries in the back of a car…asking if she worked at New Hanover Regional. She said yes and told me I looked familiar. And I said I am Zack Mayo's mom.

And she hugged me. Tight. And I told her I would never forget her kindness and thanked her for all that she did for Zack and for our family. And she shared some of her life with me. And we hugged some more. And I know God put us together. Not just in that Emergency Room—but in that parking lot **at that very moment.** And two grown women, who barely know one another—bound together by the memory of a boy loved—stand hugging tearfully, sharing life and death in a Harris Teeter parking lot.

And I return home—car full of groceries. Heart full of joy.

And I whisper a thank you to Him.

Grateful that I didn't miss an opportunity to say thank you to Karine.

Who will you thank today?

Excerpted from http://amomentatatime. org/2013/01/02/thank-you-in-a-parking-lot/[2]

That's what we do in healthcare. We make those types of differences.

My message is that I hope you recognize—and get recognized for—all the great work you do, no matter where you are in healthcare.

Every person in healthcare is significant. Don't underestimate the difference you make, even when you don't hear it, because you've answered a calling. And the calling is something that makes a difference in the lives of everybody each and every moment.

One of the nicest stories I've heard was from a CEO who shared with me that he was starting to really dig deep into the organization on who makes a difference. One day he was having a meeting with a group of people and he talked about reward and recognition. He said he was amazed that everyone kept bringing up this one person's name. John was a transporter. And he would notice that sometimes the people he was transporting were cold—especially their feet. So John carried around extra socks and he would give a pair to these patients. He had been doing this for a long, long time.

Hearing this made a big impression on the CEO. He felt that it was just so overwhelming that John cared enough to do this small act of kindness, which actually had a huge impact. He shared how in awe he is of the staff, as we all are.

I've always asked people to not assume that everyone knows the great work that is going on in your organization. Don't assume that people are aware of who's doing it. When you spot great work being done, send a note to someone in the C-suite. I guarantee you they will be grateful and will follow up.

The Power of Storytelling

I have shared several stories about the impact healthcare workers make on people's lives. You are one of those difference-makers.

Organizations have become so good at sharing the great work being done by their team. Storytelling helps everyone in the organization stay connected to the difference being made—which, in turn, keeps them tied to that crucial sense of passion and purpose. It's a great way to showcase how the organization is living its mission.

Stories are how humans have communicated since the beginning of time. Ever since humans sat around fires in caves, stories have been an important part of the way we communicate.

When we tell a story, we take a single, important moment in time and give it a multiplier effect. A story is like a single pebble tossed in a pond, rippling outward and touching others in its sphere.

Stories are tools for helping people understand and process change. They're a great way to learn and transfer knowledge.

Stories are how we remember things. When we can unite an idea with an emotion, we create something memorable for people, something that can be repeated.

The right story, well told, reconnects people to their passion in a way that other communication simply can't do. It helps lighten the load on days when our teams are weary. It rejuvenates us. Such a story can be a huge motivator.

Storytelling is a way of engaging people on a whole new level. It helps people grasp the nuances of life, not through a practical lens, but on a heart-and-soul level. It turns a message into a personal and emotional experience.

When you tell a great story, you spark a connection. We love stories because we often see ourselves in them and this helps us find commonality with others. Stories build a sense of community. We are all in this together.

Finally, stories help promote the legacy of your organization and the great people who have passed through the halls. Collecting and telling stories about the heroes on your team is a way you can thank them and honor them for the work they do.

Stories are how fire starters pass the flame to the next person. They are how we replenish that sense of calling that keeps us all going when times are tough.

In Eckhart Tolle's book *The Power of Now*, he writes, "When a log that has only just started to burn is placed next to one that is burning fiercely, and after a while they are separated again, the first log will be burning with much greater intensity. After all, it is the same fire."[3]

Stories are truly the energy that can help you reignite the passion in others. If you are the one burning fiercely, seek out those who need the spark. Share the stories of those who have made a great difference. You never know whose life you'll change for the better. You never know who needed that reminder of the calling that brought them to this place.

CHAPTER 28

A Final Word

None of this stuff is easy. Even the things we think will be easy turn out not to be. As a new leader, I really struggled with skills like communication, alignment, accountability, rewarding staff, physician engagement, and patient experience...all sound so much easier than they are. I was scared to death that I would fail, and sometimes I did.

Yet healthcare is a family, and we get through things together. I was fortunate enough to have wonderful people to lean on and learn from in the early years and in all the years since. It is thanks to them that I was able to learn what worked and what didn't so we could make some changes that made a difference. Actually, the idea for this book came from meeting and learning from so many wonderful people these many years.

My life lesson during these last few years is that a calling is not about a certain job. I find that people in healthcare answer the call at work, at home, and in their community. For me personally, I have found that a person's calling does not end when their job ends or even when their company sells. It is deeper than that. It is the intrinsic desire to make the world a better place. To all you fire starters, it is that hard-to-define DNA that requires us to respond in full when we can be helpful. The calling is a gift. It pulls us to seek solutions and to answer the call for help. To keep this gift, we must use it to benefit others. As the lyrics to "The Calling" say, "I just thank God I was listening when I got the call."

As I close writing this book, it is with a feeling of immense gratitude. When one has a full heart of gratitude, there is little room for other things. It is hard to be grateful and unhappy at the same time. These are two sayings I am drawn to.

One of the most-read columns I have ever written was about lessons from my father. One of these lessons is to do your best to make those you are with feel special. My father made anyone he met feel like they were the best part of his day. From him I learned the importance of sending letters and notes to people expressing your love and appreciation. The last letter my father was writing when he died started with "to a wonderful son." Another lesson I learned from him was to choose work that you are passionate about, because when you do, it is not work.

One of my very best friends passed away on June 30, 2019. His name was John Myslak. He had just turned 54 and he left a wonderful family behind. I spoke with John often. As his passing became closer, I spent time with him. In the last days of his life, he shared that he hated that he was dying. However, he was grateful that he had time to tell many people he loved them. He said, "Quint, make sure you tell people you love them."

Since that day, I have done so. It is interesting that the more people I express love to, the more love I feel. Most take it well. Many say it back, and a few take a bit of time to respond.

I was with Mark Clement at a TriHealth Board of Trustees meeting. Usually, we would chat while I waited for a car to pick me up and take me to the airport. Mark and I are very close; however, this day I added something. As my ride pulled up, I looked at Mark and said, "I love you." Seeing how at the time we had known each other for

27 years and I had never said these words, it was not unexpected for Mark to be taken aback. He responded with, "Your Uber is here." A few weeks later, I received a lovely handwritten note from Mark saying he loved me too.

My cousin Al says what people want most in life is to be able to love and to be loved. For many years, I was incapable of either. Today that is not the case.

Being touched by so many in healthcare who have read my books, talked with me at conferences, worked with me, and connected in various ways provides me with the feeling of being loved.

Readers, I know you realize how much I love you. I love the work you do, the difference you make, and the lives you touch. I love the way each of you responds to challenges. I love the way you are always looking to learn. I love how you forgive as well as embrace each other. I love you for being you. Thank you for answering the calling.

We Are All Fire Starters

If you ever attended one of the Studer Group Taking You and Your Organization to the Next Level conferences, you heard music. I love music. Even though I am deaf in one ear and cannot hear stereo or surround sound, music has always touched me. If you read the Introduction at the front of this book, you will have some insight into how this came to be.

As a reminder, I met singer Lisa Carrie at a Nashville workshop, and she introduced me to the accomplished musician and songwriter Alex Call. I ended up submitting some of my lyrics and they used them on a CD titled *Passion & Purpose*. One of the songs Alex, Lisa, and I collaborated on was "The Calling." (See the Introduction for the lyrics.)

Alex read my book *Hardwiring Excellence* and was moved by the section in the Conclusion called "Brian's Story." This is about my nephew who was killed in a car accident on December 24, 1995. Brian played on the University of Illinois at Chicago baseball team. Their mascot is the Flames. I did a eulogy. My message was that we can carry Brian's flame with us each day to make the world a better place.

Here is another piece of the backstory. Six months earlier, I had been keynoting a conference for the first time. The person introducing me explained that in earliest civilization, all people had important roles in their village. They were all dependent on each other for the village to survive. (This is still true today, as everyone serves an important role in the workplace and the community.) He shared that one of the roles was that of fire starter. These were people who kept the fire alive. They even had to move the fire carefully as the village moved to find game. He mentioned that at times there were storms, and the fire starters had to keep the fire alive even through these challenges.

He said that healthcare too has storms. We face choppy water, strong winds, and other threats. He added that healthcare workers need to keep the fire alive in ourselves and each other. We need fire starters. He then said, "Quint Studer is a fire starter."

Startled by the introduction, my first impulse was to push back. But then as I walked on the stage, it hit me: It was time for me to stand up and take more responsibility. I said, "Thank you. I want to be a fire starter. And I know there are many fire starters in healthcare." It caught on. At a conference, a person brought several pins in the shape of a flame. People began wearing them. People today will write to me that they are fire starters.

After Alex read *Hardwiring Excellence*, he went into the studio and recorded the song "I Can Start a Fire," which he, Lisa, and I had collaborated on. The lyrics are below. The message is that we must each do our best to keep our own internal flame bright and pass along our fire to others. Also, at times we will have our internal flame ignited by others.

We are all fire starters who have answered the calling. When healthcare gets better, the world gets better. We are all in this together.

I Can Start a Fire
(Quint Studer, Alex Call, Lisa Carrie)

This is my song
But it's not about me
It's about caring, passion, and giving
In this difficult world
What can one person do
Whoa

I can start a fire
I can keep the flame alive
I can build it higher and higher and higher
I can start a fire
Whoa, yes I can

I knew a young man
Who had to leave this life
Why was he called
Why was he called
Why am I still alive
And in his name
This is what I can do
Whoa

I can start a fire
I can keep the flame alive
I can build it higher and higher and higher
I can start a fire

Where there's only been darkness
The spark can leap from heart to heart
And I can make a difference in my own way

Maybe someday I'll hear you say
I can start a fire

And I will
And I will

Let me tell you
I can start a fire
I can keep the flame alive
I can build it higher and higher and higher
In my mind
I can start a fire
I can start a fire
Yes, I can
I can keep the flame alive
I can start a fire
I can start a fire
Oh
I can keep the flame alive
Everybody sing it now
I can start a fire
I can start a fire
I can keep the flame alive
I can keep the flame alive
I can start a fire
Oh yeah
I can keep the flame alive
And I will
Gonna start a fire
I'm burnin', burnin' in my heart
Yeah
And I will
Gonna start a fire[1]

"Legacy is not leaving something *for* people.
It's leaving something *in* people."

—Peter Strople

Thank You to Reviewers

Though my name is on the front cover, this book has truly been a group effort. Each person I have met over these many years contributed to this book. I also like to send an early version of my manuscripts to people working in the field to get their feedback. They always make it so much better, and I am so very grateful to these folks for their time, thoughtfulness, and insights. The feedback will also lead to additional tools that will be added to the website.

Jeanna Bamburg; Kevin Barnes; Keith J. Benson; Frank Borgers; Frank D. Byrne, MD; David Callecod; Dan Collard; Don Dean; Jerry Egan; Dennis Franks; Leonard H. Friedman; Marie Geissele; Dan Gentry; Shelly Gompf; Susan Knowles; Maureen Walsh Koricke; Sandi Lane; Joseph Nicosia; Kevin Post, DO; Scott Remington; Dan Springer; Anthony Stanowski; Kevin J. Valadares; Zack Ward; Dawn Zell Wright

References

Introduction

1. Call, Alex, Quint Studer, and Lisa Carrie. "The Calling." *Passion & Purpose*. Studer, 2008.

Chapter 8

1. Heath, Chip, and Dan Heath. *Switch: How to Change Things When Change Is Hard.* Broadway Books, 2010.

2. Ibid.

Chapter 9

1. Bower, Sharon Anthony, and Gordon H. Bower. *Asserting Yourself: A Practical Guide for Positive Change.* Da Capo Press, 1991.

Chapter 11

1. Curtiss, Paul R., and Phillip W. Warren. *The Dynamics of Life Skills Coaching.* Life Skills Series. Prince Albert, Saskatchewan: Training Research and Development Station, Department of Manpower and Immigration, 1973.

Chapter 13

1. Shenkar, Oded. "Defend Your Research: Imitation Is More Valuable Than Innovation." *Harvard Business Review.* April 2010. https://hbr.org/2010/04/defend-your-research-imitation-is-more-valuable-than-innovation.

Chapter 15

1. "Cal Ripken Jr. Stats." *Baseball Reference*, Sports Reference, https://www.baseball-reference.com/players/r/ripkeca01.shtml#all_br-salaries.

Chapter 16

1. Heath, Chip, and Dan Heath. *Switch: How to Change Things When Change Is Hard.* Broadway Books, 2010.

Chapter 19

1. Studer, Quint. *Hardwiring Excellence: Purpose, Worthwhile Work, Making a Difference.* Fire Starter Publishing, 2003.

Chapter 24

1. Adkins, Amy, and Brandon Rigoni. "Millennials Want Jobs to Be Development Opportunities." *Workplace.* Gallup, June 30, 2016. https://www.gallup.com/workplace/236438/millennials-jobs-development-opportunities.aspx.

Chapter 27

1. Studer, Quint. *Hardwiring Excellence: Purpose, Worthwhile Work, Making a Difference.* Fire Starter Publishing, 2003.

2. Studer, Quint. *A Culture of High Performance: Achieving Higher Quality at a Lower Cost.* Fire Starter Publishing, 2013.

3. Tolle, Eckhart. *The Power of Now: A Guide to Spiritual Enlighten-ment.* New World Library, 2004.

We Are All Fire Starters

1. Call, Alex, Quint Studer, and Lisa Carrie. "I Can Start a Fire." *Passion & Purpose.* Studer, 2008.

About the Author

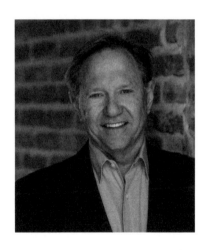

Quint Studer has spent nearly four decades in healthcare. He worked for multiple healthcare systems, the last stop being president of Baptist Hospital in Pensacola, Florida. In 2000, he founded Studer Group®, a healthcare and education coaching company. The company was sold in 2015, and Studer left in 2016. He went on to found the Studer Community Institute, a not-for-profit whose mission is to improve the quality of life for people. He has authored many books, with several listed on bestseller lists. He serves on several healthcare boards and is a frequent speaker, workshop facilitator, and mentor to individuals and organizations. The tools and techniques Quint has created over the years are now staples in healthcare systems throughout the world.

Gratitude List

Gratitude List

Gratitude List

Gratitude List

Gratitude List

Gratitude List

Gratitude List

Gratitude List